Planning for Uncertainty

David John Doukas, M.D.

William Reichel, M.D.

Planning for Uncertainty

A Guide to Living Wills and
Other Advance Directives
for Health Care

The Johns Hopkins University Press
Baltimore and London

Note to the reader: This book has been written to help the reader make decisions about his or her values relating to medical care and other issues pertaining to the quality of life. This book is not meant to substitute for the advice of medical professionals or legal counsel, and neither medical nor legal decisions should be based solely on its contents.

The authors and publisher acknowledge the assistance of Barbara Mishkin, J.D., who served as legal consultant on this project.

The Johns Hopkins University Press
2715 North Charles Street
Baltimore, Maryland 21218-4319
The Johns Hopkins Press Ltd., London

LIBRARY OF CONGRESS CATALOGING-IN-PUBLICATION DATA

Doukas, David John.
    Planning for uncertainty : a guide to living wills and other advance directives for health care / David John Doukas and
    William Reichel.
        p.   cm.
    Includes index.
    ISBN 0-8018-4670-6 (acid-free paper). — ISBN 0-8018-4671-4
    (acid-free paper : pbk.)
    1. Right to die—United States. 2. Medical care—Law and legislation—United States. 3. Power of attorney—United States. 4. Patients—Legal status, laws, etc.—United States.
    I. Reichel, William, 1937– . II. Title.
    KF3827.E87D68   1993
    344.73'04197—dc20
    [347.3044197]   93-222

A catalog record for this book is available from the British Library.

To my mentor and colleague *Laurence B. McCullough,* who kindled in me the fire to enter the field of medical ethics.   **D.J.D.**

To my son *Ralph,* whose pain and suffering has given me a glimpse into the mystery and wonder of life. He will be remembered always.   **W.R.**

Contents

Preface

As family physicians committed to the idea that patients have a right to express their preferences in medical care, we're glad you're reading this book. You've probably already recognized the importance of learning more about advance directives for medical care. We hope that this book will help you make decisions about your health care and inspire you to take action to ensure that your preferences are followed should you become unable to state your wishes.

We have both seen many, many instances in which a simple statement of medical care preferences or the designation of an alternate decision maker has prevented undue, unwanted medical hardship on a patient and needless sorrow for the family. And, sadly, we have also seen many cases in which the lack of such a document caused family members great anguish and caused the patient to suffer needlessly. As a result, we felt compelled to write a book explaining advance directives and their importance.

We can't overemphasize the fact that our experience tells us that you need to make such preparations *now.* No one ever knows when the time of need might arrive. We all know that death will come, but none of us knows exactly when. We wrote this book for everyone who wants to plan ahead for this time.

In the Introduction that follows we provide an overview of advance directive decision making in health care and discuss why and how to prepare an advance directive. We also discuss the law that has recently generated so much of the publicity about advance directives: the Patient Self-Determination Act. Chapter 1 provides more information about the background and implications of this act.

In chapter 2, we describe our concept of the difference between beneficial medical care and therapy that is futile. In chapter 3, we explore how ethical principles may conflict when health care decisions are made. Chapter 4 explains how you might go about exploring your own values regarding when to continue—and when to refuse—medical care.

Chapter 5 discusses in detail the use of the living will and the durable power of attorney for health care. Chapter 6 takes up the subject of an innovative document called the Values History, which combines the virtues of values, the living will, and the durable power of attorney for health care. The implications of family cooperation and interference in your future medical care are discussed in chapter 7. Chapter 8 examines many issues related to advance directives and explains how to complete the advance directive forms.

In the Appendix you will find information on how to obtain copies of the durable power of attorney for health care and the living will, as well as generic forms for the durable power of attorney for health care, the living will, and the Values History.

Our hope is that the information in this book will allow you to make an informed decision about advance directives, so that you can confidently face future medical situations.

Acknowledgments

This book represents the experience of the two physicians and the journey they have taken in their profession. We have each had intense experience in our work in family practice, internal medicine, geriatrics, and medical ethics. We are especially grateful to our patients, whose life stories have been the single greatest educational lesson for us as physicians.

We also want to express heartfelt acknowledgment of our editor, Jacqueline Wehmueller, who has been deeply influential in the development of this book: when it was simply a proposal, when it was being written, and upon completion of the text. It was fortuitous that she had somewhere acquired a deep and broad knowledge of advance directives. She always asked questions about the stated wishes of children in case they were stricken with a terminal illness, or about the legal status of advance directives in the mentally retarded and mentally ill. We never asked her where she acquired her insight and knowledge, or why she was so intensely interested in this project. Whatever these reasons, we are most grateful for her contributions; this book is much enriched because Jacqueline Wehmueller was our editor.

Finally, we want to refer to our personal journeys through life. The events and experiences that we have each encountered have given direction to our work. Most of all we want to thank our families—our wives, Jeanne and Helen; our children, Caitlin and Alexander Doukas and Robert and Andrea Reichel; and our parents—who were understanding and supportive while we wrote this book. We are grateful for their love, support, and graciousness, which allowed us to maintain our purpose and bring this work to fruition.

Planning for Uncertainty

Introduction: What Every Person Needs to Know

What is an advance directive?

An advance directive is an oral or written statement that tells a health care professional or health care team what forms of medical care a person would accept or would refuse in a specific medical circumstance or, alternatively, who should make health care decisions if the person is unable to express his or her own wishes. Advance directives should be in writing, although in some situations, previous statements about treatment preferences will be honored even if they were not made in writing. Moreover, a written record can clearly state what the person wants, eliminating the possibility of uncertainty, confusion, or misinterpretation. Furthermore, in some states, only by a *written* directive may certain kinds of life-sustaining treatment be refused.

Advance directives can address a wide variety of issues. They can appoint a decision-maker who will have legal power to speak for an incapacitated patient, and they can be specific, addressing particular medical therapies that the person wants or wishes to refuse. Alternatively, advance directives can be broad, providing a blanket refusal of life-sustaining medical therapy in cases of terminal illness or irreversible coma (as in a living will).

Why is an advance directive important to me?

An advance directive is important for every adult who is competent and able to make decisions about his or her future health care. First, it is easier to make decisions when you are healthy and are able to think more objectively about these topics. While some people may find thinking about these topics distressing, we know from experience that it's better to put some thought into these matters when you're well than to wait until you become sick. This is because making decisions about medical care is far more likely to be difficult for a sick person. And sometimes people are too sick to be able to make these decisions at all.

Second, if you *don't* make an advance directive and later become unable to speak for yourself, your doctor and your family may have difficulty making decisions about your care. When faced with the option that other people may have to make decisions about their care some day, most people prefer to make their own medical decisions, based on their own wishes, which can be carried out later should they become ill. Advance directives allow people to make their own choices about health care *in advance,* even though the document may be enacted when they are too sick to voice their wishes any longer.

Third, some forms of advance directives spare the family from the task of making decisions for a family member who is unable to communicate. An advance directive lifts this burden from the family—it removes a task that might otherwise be heavily laden with guilt. The benefit of such forward thinking for your own family becomes very clear. Of course, the agency of durable power of attorney may be assigned to a family member or friend who is informed about and understands your preferences, values, and beliefs.

Why do I need to think about this *now*?

Even if you are in good health, you should think about medical advance directive decision making now.

Procrastination is a common human failing: We put off doing household chores, preparing our taxes, and making out our will for the disposition of our financial estate. As physicians, we have seen the unfortunate results of procrastinating about advance directives, and we must say that the results can be devastating.

Advance directives allow you to make a decision about what kinds of health care you want in the future. You can always change your mind and alter or revoke an advance directive later. If you think about this *now*, though, and you make a decision about it *now*, and you document your decision *now*, that decision will more likely be respected and be acted upon later by your health care team.

If an advance directive is so important, why doesn't everyone have one?

Despite the importance of advance directives in health care, only a small proportion (fewer than 1 in 5) of adults have executed an advance directive. Most people haven't considered executing an advance directive because most people haven't thought (or don't wish to think) about prolonged incapacity or the end of their life. It is much easier for us to think about the "here and now" than it is to think about what prolonged incapacity or the end of our own life will be like. Many people haven't signed an advance directive because they don't know enough about it or don't know how to get one.

This book not only will explain advance directives but also will relate how easy it is to obtain an advance directive and fill it out. You can get an advance directive from your family doctor, local health department, state representative, or hospital admissions office. Private organizations such as Choice in Dying and the American Association for Retired Persons (see the Appendix) can also provide you with one.

More older people than younger people have executed an advance directive. And people are more likely to do so as they get older. Should people wait, then, until they are older to sign an advance directive? We don't think so. There's no way to predict when a serious accident or illness might occur, so it is prudent to make such plans now. Remember that the Karen Ann Quinlan and Nancy Cruzan cases involved young women, who were only in their twenties. When these young women went into a persistent vegetative state, their parents were forced to make difficult decisions about their care.

An advance directive allows you to voice your preferences regarding what sorts of things you would not want done, and what things you would want done, under specific circumstances. It also allows you to designate the person who should make treatment decisions for you in case you are not able to choose for yourself at the time a health care decision is needed. While most people find this intuitively to be a good idea, the factors of procrastination and lack of understanding probably explain why so many people have not filled out an advance directive. Some people delay signing an advance directive because they believe that they would need to pay a lawyer to help them. But neither the living will nor the durable power of attorney for health care requires the involvement of an attorney.

What role can my physician play in preparing an advance directive?

We believe that you should review your values and preferences with your personal physician before signing an advance directive (see chapter 5). The ideal is for everyone to have a personal physician and to hold conversations with that physician. For all those who don't enjoy continuity of care with a personal physician, we believe that being in an ongoing, trusting doctor-patient relationship is a shared responsibility for patients and the health care system. A discussion with your physician will give you some insight into the consequences of the many decisions that can be made about medical care. By discussing these matters with your personal doctor, you will have a much better understanding of what you are consenting to or refusing, and why. Signing an advance directive after careful thought and informed discussion is obviously preferable to signing with little reflection or understanding. Also, as a result of these discussions, your personal physician will have a much better understanding of your motivations and feelings.

What is a living will?

A living will is a declaration or statement allowing a person to direct that life-sustaining medical therapies be withdrawn or withheld in the future if the person is terminally ill and no longer able to make decisions. Living wills are currently recognized by statute in all but three states (the exceptions are Massachusetts, Michigan, and New York). In a few states, living wills also apply to persons in a persistently vegetative state. (The terms *terminal illness* and *persistently vegetative state* are discussed in chapter 5.) A "generic" living will can be helpful in those states where the living will has not yet been recognized by statute (see the Appendix). A living will can tell your doctor and your family your preferences regarding life-sustaining therapies, so they have a basis upon which to act if you can no longer speak for yourself.

A living will, therefore, is a written advance directive. It allows you to put in writing your wish not to have life-sustaining medical therapies begun or continued if you are dying from a terminal illness. It does *not* allow you to demand treatment that would not benefit you.

What is a durable power of attorney?

The durable power of attorney gives someone you designate the legal authority to act or make decisions on your behalf. The *durable* aspect of this document is important, because without provisions making a power of attorney durable, a (simple) power of attorney will become void when the person who wrote it becomes incapacitated. That is, a *power of attorney* recognizes the authority of one person to act or make decisions only for another *competent* person. A *durable power of attorney* recognizes the authority of one person to act or make decisions for an *incompetent* person. To be *durable,* the power of attorney must include a provision similar to one of the following:

1. This power of attorney shall not be affected by my incapacity; or
2. This power of attorney will take effect upon my incapacity.

The durable power of attorney is recognized in every state and the District of Columbia. In addition, some states have laws more specifically addressing durable powers of attorney for health care.

What is a durable power of attorney for health care?

A durable power of attorney for health care is a document delegating authority to another person to make decisions *specifically about health care.* It allows you to transfer your authority to whomever you choose, so that he or she will decide which medical therapies to accept and which to refuse if you are unable to speak for yourself. It also allows you to state your preferences regarding future medical care, so that if someday you are unable to communicate, the person speaking for you has instructions from you about what you want done or not done. (A generic durable power of attorney for health care form can be found in the Appendix)

A durable power of attorney for health care is different from other durable powers of attorney in that it specifically addresses only *health care issues.* Importantly, it does not give anyone authority to manage the person's estate or to make financial decisions. It is our understanding that every state that recognizes the durable power of attorney recognizes a durable power of attorney for health care, with the apparent exception of Oklahoma, whose attorney general in 1991 wrote an opinion expressing his view that health care decision making cannot be delegated from one person to another person.

What is a proxy?

A proxy, also known as an *agent,* or *health care surrogate,* is the person selected to serve as an agent under a durable power of attorney for health care. The proxy has the power to make medical decisions for the patient when he or she is unable to do so. The proxy uses his or her understanding of the patient's values and preferences regarding various medical therapies to make decisions about treatment. This understanding is based on previous conversations and written advance directives. The decisions made by the proxy should reflect the decisions the patient would have made, given the medical circumstances under consideration, if he or she had been able to. The proxy should, of course, also follow any written instructions provided by the patient in the durable power of attorney for health care, or in any other document.

If I sign an advance directive, how long will it remain in effect?

Any advance directive you sign when competent will remain in effect unless or until you revoke it. *Only you can revoke your own advance directive.* You can do so by crossing out parts of or completely destroying your current advance directive. Or you can sign and date a new advance directive and make it clear that it replaces any others you have signed in the past. You can do this whenever you wish. This revocation is allowed in many states even if you are no longer competent.

1

What the Patient Self-Determination Act Means to You

What is the Patient Self-Determination Act?

Passed by Congress late in 1990, the Patient Self-Determination Act (PSDA) is a federal law that took effect on December 1, 1991. It requires all hospitals, nursing homes, home health agencies, hospices, and health maintenance organizations that receive Medicare or Medicaid funds to provide patients with a written statement of their rights under state law to accept or refuse treatment and to prepare advance directives for health care. The Patient Self-Determination Act also requires these institutions to ask patients if they have signed an advance directive, and it prohibits discrimination against patients on the basis of whether or not they have signed an advance directive. In some facilities, living will and durable power of attorney forms may be available to patients, and signed advance directives may be photocopied and placed in the medical record. The medical system of the

Veterans Administration is expected to follow suit shortly with its own version of the Act's requirements.

The Patient Self-Determination Act may become a powerful new force that will encourage patients to consider writing advance directives. At the same time, the Patient Self-Determination Act, we hope, will encourage all persons to make these arrangements when they are *well, before* they become patients.

Why did Congress pass the Patient Self-Determination Act?

Originally, the authors of the Patient Self-Determination Act hoped that it would help achieve the passage of advance directive legislation in all states. The Congress passed the Patient Self-Determination Act in order to educate physicians, nurses, health care administrators, and consumers about advance directives. Thus, Congress hoped the law would result in increased citizen awareness of the living will and the durable power of attorney for health care.

Part of the stimulus for the introduction of this legislation was the unfortunate case of Nancy Cruzan. This prominent case dealt with a very difficult situation involving a request to withdraw a feeding tube from a young woman who was in a persistent vegetative state (this case is discussed in chapter 8). The public debate evoked by this case helped to stimulate congressional concern about advance directives, as well.

What is the Patient Self-Determination Act supposed to do?

The Patient Self-Determination Act is intended to ensure that all patients are made aware of their rights concerning health care and advance directive decisions at the time of admission to hospitals and other health care settings. The Act affords patients an opportunity, if they wish, to prepare an advance directive before they become incompetent or unable to do so. The Patient Self-Determination Act is meant to provide an opportunity for the patient to learn about and prepare instructions about health care (advance directives) in case they might be needed later.

When did the law take effect?

The Patient Self-Determination Act took effect on December 1, 1991, throughout the United States. If you have been hospitalized since then, you should have been asked about advance directives when you were being admitted.

How does it work?

According to the Patient Self-Determination Act, all patients being admitted to a health care institution that receives Medicare or Medicaid funds will be given written information about their legal rights regarding advance directives and the institution's policies for honoring those rights. This process is to take place at the time of admission, unless the patient's condition makes it impracticable. Materials on the institution's advance directives policy must also be provided. In addition, the patient (or the patient's legal representative) must be asked during the admissions process whether he or she already has signed an advance directive. If the patient requests specific materials on living wills and durable powers of attorney, such information may be available from the institution's counsel or administration.

If it is not an emergency when a patient is admitted to the hospital, the admissions clerk (or possibly a social worker or nurse) may give the patient a written statement describing the health care institution's obligations to honor patients' health care requests, including advance directives. (Indeed, we believe it is unfortunate that there is no mandate for these discussions to be initiated by the patient's physician.)

If the patient has signed a living will or durable power of attorney, this fact must be entered into the patient's medical record. Hospitals typically enter copies of advance directives into the patient's medical record when the patient has signed one—in fact, most states' advance directive laws *require* that a copy of the signed advance directive be placed in the patient's record. If an advance directive has not been signed by the patient, he or she may request the written materials needed to sign an advance directive (these usually are available to the patient).

In other circumstances (when a patient enters the hospital in an emergency and is unconscious, for example), the first concern is to provide medical care. In such an event, the designated person would provide the hospital's advance directive policy materials to the patient's proxy or family (if they have accompanied the patient) and ask if the patient has signed an advance directive. If so, a copy of the advance directive may be placed in the patient's medical record. The facility is still obliged to approach the patient with these materials when he or she is medically stable and is no longer incapacitated.

In reality, this could become an automatic and trivialized process. For example, when a patient is admitted to the hospital, the admissions clerk might ask whether he or she has a living will or durable power of attorney. If the clerk merely accepts an affirmative response and enters this information into the record and gives the patient a policy sheet on advance directives before moving on, certain important issues have not been addressed. The location of the advance directive (accessibility is crucial) and the naming of an agent through a durable power of attorney agent (location and willingness of the agent are important) are pieces of information that could be overlooked. Merely asking if you have an advance directive may not be enough.

Also, if interactions with health professionals following admission do not result in the mention or discussion of advance directives at all, the patient may not have an adequate opportunity to convey the intent of his or her directive. We believe that the Patient Self-Determination Act should not only facilitate communication with patients about their consent or refusal of medical treatments, but also result in a discussion of the meaning of these decisions with a health professional.

Further, under the Patient Self-Determination Act, these health care institutions have an obligation to train their staff and educate the public concerning the options of advance directive use. Unfortunately, as in certain other pieces of legislation that Congress has passed, no money was allocated to cover the expense of these educational efforts or the distribution of advance directives to patients. Indeed, since no special training was mandated specifically for members of the health care staff providing the patient with information, quality control for the process of informing patients has been a concern. Nevertheless, hospitals and other health agencies appear to be doing their best to carry out the Patient Self-Determination Act mandate, despite the additional time and money required.

A final provision of the law mandates that each state develop or approve the written materials on advance directives that will be given to patients, and that the federal government develop similar materials for distribution to health professionals and beneficiaries of Social Security, while at the same time developing a national educational effort on advance directives for the general population.

Which staff member is responsible for asking the patient about advance directives?

The PSDA leaves this up to the facility. This is one of the areas of weakness of the law. We have already pointed out that the law does not mandate that physicians ask about and discuss advance directives with the patient. This role often is carried out by the admissions clerk (and in some cases by social workers or nurses). We believe that the law is relying on inpatient or institutional settings to carry out a function that should take place over a period of time in the outpatient or office setting. With the exception of the requirement of the law that applies to health maintenance organizations, the law does not encourage people to prepare an advance directive before hospitalization or nursing home placement becomes necessary. Finally, as mentioned above, by the time the person reaches the hospital or long-term facility, he or she may not be competent to discuss treatment preferences, choices, or values. These are problems that must be addressed by patients and their doctors in the next decade to improve the pioneering efforts of the Patient Self-Determination Act.

What is a Medicare- or Medicaid-receiving health care institution?

Most hospitals, nursing homes, hospices, home health agencies, and health maintenance organizations receive payments from Medicare or Medicaid. If they do, they are subject to the requirements of the Patient Self-Determination Act.

What happens if the Act is not followed?

If the hospitals or health agencies do not follow the Patient Self-Determination Act, they risk losing elegibility to receive Medicare and Medicaid payments. The Congress believes that risk provides sufficient motivation for them to comply with the Act.

Will I only be asked about advance directives if I'm being admitted to a hospital or being enrolled in a health maintenance organization?

At this time under the Patient Self-Determination Act, it is when you are being admitted to a hospital, nursing home, home health agency, or hospice, or being enrolled in a health maintenance organization that you must be asked about your advance directives. However, you might come across materials on this subject in doctors' offices, clinics, and other outpatient settings, as well. It is our hope that doctors will discuss advance directives with their patients during routine office visits.

Who else should talk with me about advance directives?

Discussions prompted by the Patient Self-Determination Act at Medicare- and Medicaid-funded facilities are not the only discussions you ought to have about advance directive options. It's a good idea to sit down with your doctor (if you have one) to discuss the advance directives that are recognized in your state. Write down what you would like to have done in the future if you are ever terminally ill or are unable to express your wishes about medical treatment. You may also be asked about advance directives when you are planning your financial estate with your attorney.

In any case, now is the appropriate time to consider filling out an advance directive, because your current interest in this topic suggests that you appreciate the wisdom of signing one, and your understanding of this subject will have been enhanced from reading this book. The more information on advance directives you have, the more informed your choices will be when you sign one. That is why we describe the types of advance directives in detail in the upcoming chapters.

Whether the Patient Self-Determination Act will someday be extended to outpatient clinics and private doctors' offices is presently unknown. In our view, such an approach would clearly be beneficial to all patients.

Is this just more admissions paperwork?

We hope not, but the potential exists. If patients are given only the minimum required information, that information may be reduced down to a few written pages that could easily be shuffled into the rest of the admissions paperwork (the consent forms and insurance information, for example).

Nothing could be more counterproductive to the spirit of the Patient Self-Determination Act than burying the patient under an avalanche of paper into which the material on advance directives is shuffled, perhaps never to be seen by the patient. To make sure this doesn't happen to you, you can learn about advance directives and fill them out now, before you have to go to a hospital or nursing home, and then take them with you if you need to go to the hospital or nursing home.

How can I make sure this law works for me?

The best way to make sure the Patient Self-Determination Act works for you is to see if the materials offered to you provoke your thought. If these materials make you reflect on advance directives, if they make you search inside yourself to decide what your wishes are and how you would like certain medical care decisions carried out, the Patient Self-Determination Act would appear to be working for you. If, instead, you are handed some sheets of paper that you don't understand, you would probably be better off speaking to a doctor, nurse, or someone else who can explain the document and help you express your wishes.

Have there been other objections raised against the Patient Self-Determination Act?

Yes, there have been several points of contention. Some have argued that the paperwork and personnel time needed to fulfill the requirements are too costly. However, one need only consider that the care of a single patient in a persistently vegetative state may cost more than $100,000 each year to realize that the investment is worthwhile. Some people have argued that advance directives are already widely available. Yet, the rate of signing has been quite low. Others have argued that it is the patient's responsibility, or that it is too uncomfortable for doctors to speak to patients about death and advance directives, or that the requirements of the Patient Self-Determination Act might upset the patient who is being admitted to the hospital or long-term facility. However, we believe that the right of the patient to give an informed consent (chapter 3) is reason enough to conform to the Act.

Some people contend that this act should only apply to the elderly and debilitated. But many people become terminally ill or have serious accidents that leave them persistently vegetative. Also, although health care institutions are prohibited under the Patient Self-Determination Act from requiring an advance directive, some people argue that the Act will coerce patients indirectly to sign advance directives, so that the health care institution will save costs surrounding end-of-life care. This concern is important, for it illustrates today's collision between cost-containment concerns in medicine and the freedom of the patient to make a decision. The intrusion of any institution into an individual's ability to consent to a therapy is ethically unacceptable to us, whether or not such intrusion profits a hospital or society as a whole.

If these objections aren't convincing, do you see any problems with this law?

In our view, the Patient Self-Determination Act *does* have shortcomings. As discussed above, for example, the Act does not require that physicians talk to patients; rather, the exchange of information can occur at the admissions desk, along with the rest of the paperwork given to the patient at this time. This lack of contact between physician and patient undermines efforts toward educating patients about advance directives and gaining their consent.

Also, outpatient medical facilities and clinics (except health maintenance organizations, hospices, and home health agencies) are not affected by the Act. Yet, patients admitted to the hospital are not optimal candidates for advance directive decision making, for they may be in pain, they may be fearful, or they may not be able to respond. We believe strongly that efforts to educate patients about advance directives should also be a priority in the outpatient health care setting. Doctors owe it to all their adult patients to routinely discuss personal choices about health care, including the choice of refusing treatment in the event of future terminal illness or incompetence, so that patients have an opportunity to voice their preferences.

What improvements might be in the offing?

The Patient Self-Determination Act could be improved in a variety of ways that might broaden its scope. Discussions with patients could be offered in all medical offices, clinics, and health care institutions. Money could be allocated to fund public service programs and programs for medical staff that would educate people about the use of advance directives. Attorneys and health insurance companies could more actively encourage the use of advance directives among their clients. All of these proposals might be given greater attention if the public demands it of legislators, attorneys, and insurance companies.

How might the law help me?

Few physicians have discussed living wills and durable powers of attorney with their patients, and few patients have signed these documents. The Patient Self-Determination Act requires health care facilities to provide education for their staff and members of the community about advance directives. In addition, people will receive information about, and have the opportunity to receive copies of, a living will and durable power of attorney for health care when they are admitted to a health care facility. If a person is offered one of these advance directives on admission, there is a much greater likelihood that the person will sign an advance directive. Family members and physicians will thereby know what the patient's treatment choices would be, given certain situations, and the patient can be confident that they will follow his or her instructions.

Only time will tell how effective the Patient Self-Determination Act will be in increasing the use of advance directives. Regardless of the impact of the Act, however, you can consider your advance directive options now, so that your preferences will be well thought through and clearly stated for others to understand and implement, if that becomes necessary. In chapter 2, we explain further why, based on our experience, we believe that an advance directive is an important document for you to consider.

2

When Is Therapy Beneficial?
When Is It Futile?

What are life-sustaining therapies?

Life-sustaining therapies are medical treatments that prolong a person's life. While life-sustaining therapies may not return you to your previous state of health, they will keep you alive. There are many kinds of treatment that are life-sustaining, including breathing machines (respirators or ventilators), feeding tubes (inserted through your nose or abdomen into your stomach), and intravenous hydration and medication (fluids given through a vein). These therapies are discussed in detail in chapter 6. In our view, life-sustaining therapy may be appropriate at certain times and not appropriate at others. We discuss below the difference between these two times.

What is heroic therapy?

Heroic therapy is a term that in the past was applied to life-sustaining therapy. Although the term has fallen into disfavor, many of our patients and colleagues, as well as the media, continue to use it. The basic premise is that the patient is undertaking a heroic and valiant effort to save him- or herself. In light of the heroic intent, the patient's attempt is supposedly seen as being worthwhile and justified. However, there are times when such therapy does not benefit the patient and therefore would not be considered "heroic," but merely life sustaining. Therefore, the term *life-sustaining therapy* is preferable to the more dated term *heroic therapy.*

What are nutrition and hydration?

Nutrition is a generic term that covers a broad range of means of providing nutrients (food or specially prepared liquid formulas) to a patient. These methods include self-provided nutrition (by mouth); nutrition provided by someone else (spoon feeding); nutrition provided by inserting a tube through the nose down to the stomach or the small intestine (a nasogastric tube), so that liquefied food can be delivered; nutrition provided by surgically inserting a tube into the stomach or into the small intestine (a gastrostomy tube), so that liquid nutrition can be supplied; and nutrition provided by putting a tube into a vein so that nutritionally simple nutrients in a liquid form can be delivered directly into the bloodstream.

Hydration is defined as providing water, often supplemented with chemicals, to maintain a proper chemical balance in the bloodstream. The use of nutrition and hydration are often collectively considered in medical decisions because their delivery goes hand in hand. They provide the necessary sustenance while the patient is unable to swallow food, and they help the patient avoid malnutrition and chemical imbalances.

Discontinuation of nutrition and hydration will inevitably lead to death. Some people feel uncomfortable about stopping nutrition and hydration because they believe that doing so is the equivalent of depriving a patient of the food and water needs that are basic and required, and that doing so will inflict suffering. (Indeed, some living will statutes exclude the withholding or withdrawal of nutrition and hydration). On the other hand, many physicians and patients believe that nutrition and hydration are like other medical therapies that patients should be entitled to refuse. This is the position taken by virtually all the courts that have considered the question, as well as by the American Medical Association.

One point needs to be made about the concern over causing pain: stopping nutrition and hydration are usually considered when the person is near the end of life or has markedly diminished mental function. The discontinuation of such therapy usually is combined with the administration of pain-relieving medications as needed, to ensure that the person feels no discomfort.

For example, consider the case of a woman with terminal cancer who has written a living will specifically requesting the discontinuation of nutrition and hydration if she becomes terminally ill and no longer is able to communicate. The actual withdrawal (that is, the removal of the various tubes from her body) may take but an instant, yet the process of the disease ending her life may take several days. During this process, efforts would be made to ensure that she does not feel discomfort from dehydration. Comfort care measures would be taken— her mouth would be moistened and she would be kept clean. Medicines would still be administered to alleviate her pain. If she became unconscious, the probability that she would perceive pain is even more remote. Taking measures to minimize the chance of her experiencing pain helps to reassure the patient's family, however, and helps to prevent suffering on the part of the patient.

Is stopping life-sustaining treatment like suicide or killing?

It is our belief that stopping life-sustaining care, when a patient is terminally ill or persistently vegetative, is not like suicide or active killing, because the withdrawal or withholding of therapy is not the cause of the person's death. (This is also the position taken by most courts and state statutes.) Rather, the therapy is merely prolonging the person's life while the disease is killing the patient.

Some people think that if they forgo the use of a ventilator or a feeding tube, they will be assisting in a form of suicide, or that if they request the cessation of such care for someone else, they will be engaging in a form of murder—but that is not the case. Forgoing therapy allows the disease to progress as it would without medical intervention. As most courts and state legislatures have stated, forgoing therapy for a terminally ill person allows life to end more naturally by letting the disease run its course.

Is stopping a therapy the same as never starting it?

Patients and their families often ask this question when they make an artificial distinction between not starting (or withholding) a therapy and stopping a therapy. The law makes no such distinction. The two options need viewing in the same light, for three reasons.

First, in considering the use of medical therapies, it is very important to find out whether a specific medical therapy will benefit the person. If a patient could never stop a therapy once started, he or she could never *try* a therapy. Placing a restriction on the use of life-sustaining therapies—that they must be continued, once started—is fallacious, because the initiation of a therapy would require its being continued indefinitely.

Second, people have a right to refuse medical therapies, and this applies to therapies already begun as well as to those yet to be initiated. Because a therapy is life-sustaining does not mean that a person cannot refuse that therapy or stop its use.

Finally, the notion that stopping a therapy is a form of suicide or killing is also fallacious, for the reasons stated above. Therefore, if the patient (or his or her proxy) wishes to stop a therapy, he or she ought to be allowed to do so. It is the illness that kills, not the person who stops the therapy.

What are benefits and burdens?

The terms *benefits* and *burdens* are often used when discussing whether or not a medical therapy should be used or discontinued. When a person considers whether a therapy is worth using, he or she first determines if the benefits gained by accepting that therapy outweigh the burdens endured by accepting that therapy.

How does a patient weigh benefits and burdens?

Benefits and burdens can't simply be quantified and then weighed against one another. The weighting of a harm or a benefit should be done from the patient's point of view. That is, the respective weight assigned to a harm and a benefit will be influenced by many factors, such as the values of the patient; the memories the patient has of his or her own past illnesses and those of his or her family and friends; and the patient's attitude toward his or her illness.

Consider the person who has a nasogastric tube (a tube passed through the nose down the esophagus to the stomach or small intestine for administration of liquid nutrition and hydration). That tube may be uncomfortable, and yet it may be the only means by which the person can stay alive. The benefit is that the person is sustained nutritionally with that tube. It is not uncommon, however, for a person who is being fed through such a tube to develop repeated pneumonias. These lung infections occur because the liquid food, after being delivered to the stomach through the tube, can back up into the esophagus (which connects the mouth to the stomach) to the windpipe, and from there into the lungs.

A person who has had repeated pneumonias from the food administered in this way may experience these infections as a burden resulting from the tube. If the person is terminally ill, the nutritional benefit of keeping the tube in place may not be worth the burden of repeated pneumonia. People who have seen a friend or family member go through a similar experience may respond to such memories by indicating that they believe the burden outweighs the potential benefit of this treatment.

What's involved in weighing benefits and burdens?

Weighing benefits and burdens is a difficult thing to do because it must be done on a case-by-case basis. Diseases differ, and so does the severity of illnesses. Not everyone values or weighs benefits and burdens in the same way. For these reasons, benefits and burdens must be weighed on an individualized basis.

Sometimes the weighing of benefits and burdens takes place between the physician and the patient's family, after the patient can no longer speak. That's one reason it's a good idea to discuss what treatment you consider burdensome with your family and your physician—so that other people will understand how you define an unbearable burden. (Such discussions may take place over an extended time, as you come to know your doctor.) Having conversations with family members can also help convey this information for use in the future, if you are ever unable to speak.

How does my notion of benefit versus burden affect my preferences?

Your definition of beneficial treatment and your definition of burdensome treatment will determine to some degree what you need to discuss with your family and with your physician. You may have strong feelings about which types of medical illness (and their degree of severity) should be treated and which types (and severity) should not be treated by any form of medical treatment. In such cases, it is best to document your beliefs in a clear-cut way in an advance directive.

The decisions you make need to be well informed, and

you also need to understand the implications of the many medical scenarios that can occur in your future. For this reason, you need to acquaint yourself with the outcomes of different types of disease. Yet, you can't be expected to predict your own future—you can only speculate on the reasonable outcomes of your current health status, with the risk factors you know about, including family disease history and your own use of tobacco, drugs, and alcohol. People with lung disease who continue to smoke cigarettes, for example, may already have decided how they feel about being placed on a ventilator (breathing machine) if their lungs suddenly stopped working.

What is futile therapy?

Futile therapy is a term for therapy that provides no medical benefit at all. In this case, the prospect of a specific medical therapy being effective is so bleak that it is considered futile to start or continue that therapy. Thus, some therapies could be considered futile even if they were not burdensome (because they don't improve the patient's condition). Therapy is considered futile if it would have no demonstrable medical benefit for this or any patient in the same situation. For someone who is in the last stages of a terminal illness, most therapies would probably be considered futile, but treatments designed to keep the patient comfortable are still valuable.

Is the doctor obliged to discuss futile therapy with a patient?

Some doctors would say no. In their view, because the therapy isn't a beneficial therapy, there is no requirement to bring it up. Other doctors say yes. Because the patient may have expectations of receiving certain therapies as his or her life is ending, these doctors reason, the patient should be informed that these therapies will not help.

Physicians should not offer a therapy if it has no benefit, but we believe they should at least explain why such therapy would not help the patient. In any event, physicians are not required to *provide* futile therapy. We believe that if there is no benefit to a therapy, the patient has no right to demand that the doctor provide it. A question remains, though:

Is futility the same for everyone?

No, it is not. In our view, the notion of futility must be related to the age and overall medical condition of the patient. The healthier the patient, the higher the expectation of recovery; hence, the lower the likelihood that medical therapies would be futile. (We discuss the impact of age and illness on medical decision making further in chapter 8.) Medical therapies that are appropriate for a young adult who has had a sudden reversible illness are much more likely to succeed than the same therapies administered to an elderly patient with multiple medical problems, chronic diseases, or terminal illness. The concept of futility is also case-specific to the patient's illness. The therapies physicians might offer a vital and healthy elder may be inappropriate for a patient of any age who is terminally ill and has, for example, a widespread bacterial infection (known as *sepsis*).

The word *futility* may *mean* very different things for the patient and the doctor, too, for their hopes for recovery are dependent on their respective expectations of outcome in the illness process. Sometimes, the patient's hopes for recovery are unrealistic and do not appropriately weigh the impact of the disease. When irrational demands are placed on a health care team to perform futile therapy, it can be very difficult for everyone involved. Some people hold on much longer than others to a last chance—for some last, best effort—to fight a disease or illness. Often, controversies surrounding the futility of therapy occur when communications between the health provider, the patient, and the family are found to be wanting. When expectations of outcome and ideas about useful (and futile) therapies differ between parties, it is not surprising that conflict occurs.

Sometimes treatment does not alleviate the state of the illness but does allow the patient hours or days of consciousness that he or she will value highly. Some people want to try to survive for the birth of a grandchild, or for the celebration of a religious holiday, or to bid farewell to a relative who is traveling to see them. Therefore, the treatment that allows continued consciousness (if it does so while eliminating pain) may be valuable to individuals even when death is unavoidable and imminent.

Will my doctor tell me if something is futile?

More than likely, your doctor will be forthright in telling you if something may be a futile therapy for you in your circumstances. On the other hand, your doctor may not believe that it is ever necessary to offer or discuss futile therapies. If you sense that this is true, you may want to have a serious talk with the doctor, to inform him or her of your desire to be kept informed of your health status, even if therapies are no longer of benefit. If your doctor is honest with you about your condition, you can prepare yourself for the time you have remaining, knowing that medical therapies will no longer be beneficial.

Sometimes doctors disagree about when the point of futility for a therapy has been reached. For instance, one doctor may believe a therapy is futile, while another may be optimistic in trying a therapy or an approach that may have some benefit but that carries a significant burden. The uses of many medications fall into this category. There may be a benefit to be gained by taking a certain drug, yet this drug therapy may have severe side effects that adversely affect the patient's quality of life. Whether your doctor considers a particular therapy futile is something you need to discuss with your doctor. Understandably, these estimations will change with your age, your severity of illness, your short-term and long-term prognosis, and the medical interventions that are available to you.

Can I request futile therapy?

You may request therapies your doctor believes to be futile, but he or she is not required to provide them. The decision will depend on how all parties concerned view that therapy. If you believe that there is a particular therapy that may help you, and if you have a reasoned understanding of what that therapy is and how it might help you, you should discuss it with your doctor. If your doctor refuses to consider your request, you have the right to ask for a second opinion. It may be that another doctor will disagree with your doctor, or it may be that you do not fully realize the severity of the disease or the futility of the treatment. Frank discussion between you and your doctor often proves a potent antidote to faulty communication.

What if my doctor refuses to provide a therapy?

The best thing to do in these circumstances is to be open and honest in your discussions with your doctor, so that your doctor understands why you are requesting the therapy. You also need to ask your doctor questions so that you understand why your doctor is making the decisions he or she is making. Everyone involved needs to understand the realistic course of the disease as well as the realistic hopes that you have of fighting that disease. If there is a certain risk in a medical therapy that you are willing to accept, then it is best to discuss that with your physician early, so that he or she knows how hard you wish to fight your illness. If there is disagreement between you and your physician over the appropriateness of a therapy, then requesting a second opinion or a referral to another physician may be an advisable course of action. Your doctor may perceive an advanced disease state as a lost war, not as an ongoing battle.

Can I *demand* futile therapy?

Demanding something *that will not benefit you* makes no medical sense, regardless of the *perceived* benefit. Perhaps the best thing to do in such circumstances is to sit down with your family and your doctor and discuss realistically what your medical options are. If you and your doctor have differing expectations regarding your medical care, it is best to address them as soon as possible.

As an example, consider an elderly man with many

medical problems who enters the hospital with chest pain and is diagnosed as having a myocardial infarction (heart attack) due to severe coronary artery disease. His doctor believes that medical management is adequate for the patient's needs, considering his advanced years, and fears that he will not survive an operation to bypass the diseased arteries to his heart. The doctor tells the patient that his survival is not expected to be more than a few more years. The doctor does not inform him of the option of undergoing bypass surgery. The patient, however, requests that he be considered for a bypass operation— "like a friend of mine just had." The doctor explains to the patient that he is not a candidate for this operation, but the patient demands (with his family's agreement) that the operation be done. The doctor refuses to perform what he perceives to be a futile procedure, but he volunteers the names of several doctors who might consider performing the operation. Two of the other doctors also refuse to operate; the third doctor believes that, although there is substantial risk, the operation is feasible. The operation is performed, and the patient initially does well in the surgical intensive care unit. Several hours later, however, the patient's heart arrests (stops) and cardiopulmonary resuscitation is performed. The patient's heart is restarted but he never regains consciousness.

One week later, the doctor explains to the family that the patient is in an irreversible comatose state, that his chances of recovery to a thinking state are nonexistent, and that the doctor has placed a "no code" order on the chart. A *no code order* means that no attempts will be made to restart the heart or lungs if in the future they fail to function. The family is adamantly against this order and demands that it be removed from the chart. The doctor states that a code would be futile treatment, and that he is willing to facilitate the transfer of the patient to another doctor. The doctor points out to the family that the patient's state is grave and asks the family if the patient would want to be resuscitated in his current state, with no hope of recovery. The family discusses this aspect of the patient's values and decides that he would not want such attempts made if, in the end, he would be incompetent and unable to think and speak. After these discussions among themselves and with the doctor, the family agrees to keep the no code order on the chart. The patient dies the next day, after suffering another heart attack.

In this example, the patient, the patient's family, and the health care providers all had to make decisions based on their understanding of the possible benefits and futility of the situation and on their beliefs, or values, as well as on the ethical principles involved. In chapter 3, we discuss the ethical principles that influence health care decisions.

3

How Ethical Principles Affect Health Care Decisions

What is autonomy?

Autonomy is the ethical principle describing the right to self-determination, including the right to be left alone and to make your own decisions without interference from other people. It is also the basis for your doctor's responsibility to respect your decisions about medical care, confidentiality, and refusal of care. The principle of autonomy is rooted in several concepts, including social notions of individual freedom, constitutional rights of liberty and privacy, and U.S. court decisions made over the past several decades.

What is beneficence?

Beneficence is the principle that gives force to the physician's responsibility to attempt to benefit the patient medically while attempting to minimize harm to the patient. The foundations of this principle are over 2,500 years old, reaching back to the time of Hippocrates, when physicians were encouraged to treat their patients while being mindful of not harming them in the process.

Why are these principles of concern to me?

These principles are of concern to you—indeed, they are of concern to us all—because they address your ability to make decisions as well as your expectation that information will be given to you so you can make those decisions (within the autonomy principle), and because the physician has a responsibility to do his or her best to try to benefit you and protect you from harm (within the beneficence principle).

The doctor's beneficence-based duties toward the patient occasionally conflict with the patient's autonomy. Physicians are sometimes *paternalistic* (that is, excessively beneficent), so that they insist on helping patients whether the patient wants the help or not. While they may have good intentions, physicians who act paternalistically may violate the dignity and rights of the patient.

Paternalistic behavior can restrict your decision-making autonomy in various ways. If the doctor were to withhold information from you to "spare" you anguish, or if you were forced to accept a certain treatment plan because your doctor did not inform you of available alternatives, or if, in the extreme, the physician forced a therapy upon you through coercive means, your freedom to decide would be diminished. Such behavior is professionally unethical and probably illegal.

Let's consider the example of a young woman who is

diagnosed as having thyroid cancer and is sent to a surgeon who tells her that the tumor and surrounding tissue need to be removed. In response to the patient's question about risks, the surgeon plays down the risks of infection and bleeding and does not even mention the resulting scar and the risk of injury to the nerves going to both sides of the vocal cords. Not wanting to worry the patient, the doctor hides this information from her. After surgery, the patient discovers that one of the two nerves to the vocal cords is irreparably severed during the procedure, leaving her with speech difficulties; further, she is upset by the appearance of the scar on her neck.

This case raises the question of whether the patient would have agreed to undergo the surgery had these outcomes been explained to her. The point here is that the patient would, at the very least, have been able to prepare herself mentally for such a possible adverse outcome if the risks had been discussed with her and she chose to accept them. Paternalism in this case took the form of a doctor hiding something from a patient due to a desire to protect her from what the doctor perceived to be an unnecessary concern.

What do advance directives have to do with the principles of autonomy and beneficence?

Advance directives are designed to help you exercise your right to decide autonomously which medical therapies you want. When competent, you are always free to consent to or refuse any therapy. Therefore, you have a right to decide *beforehand,* that is, *before* you should become unable to speak for yourself, which therapies you want attempted and which therapies you believe aren't worthwhile to you in continuing your life. The doctor's autonomy-based obligation is to follow your preferences, and his or her beneficence-based obligation is to offer and use only those therapies that will benefit you.

What are informed consent and informed refusal?

Informed consent is a mechanism for honoring the principle of autonomy. Because of the principle of autonomy, your doctor has a duty to tell you about your medical condition, the risks and benefits of therapies that might help you, and what might happen to you if you elect to have no treatment at all (this process is called *disclosure*). Your doctor also has the responsibility to make sure that you understand all of this information (he or she must ensure *comprehension*). You must be able to make your decision without an impairing mental condition (such as psychosis or severe dementia), and without anyone trying to coerce you (for example, your doctor, a nurse, a third-party health care payer, or a family member). If you are able to understand your medical situation as well as available treatment options, and if you are *free of constraints* when you make your decision, then you are able to give informed consent.

You might also give an informed refusal. You have the autonomous right to refuse any medical therapy, and to have that refusal respected by your doctor and family, as long as you have decision-making capacity when you make this decision. The necessary components of disclosure, comprehension, and freedom from constraints apply to refusal, just as they do to consent.

What questions should I ask my doctor during the informed consent phase of considering therapy?

If you are in the hospital or a doctor's office and the doctor suggests initiating a therapy for you, ask questions. Here are some examples:

What is my medical condition called?
What are the implications of this condition?
What will happen to me as time goes on?
What is my short-term prognosis? What is my long-term prognosis?
What is the therapy called?
What does the therapy do?
How does the therapy work?
How invasive is the therapy?
How long will I have to continue the therapy?
What is the benefit to be gained by using this therapy?
What are the risks of this therapy?
What other therapies may possibly be beneficial to me?
What would happen if I didn't treat my condition?
What are the chances this therapy will help me?
Will I (or my proxy) be free to stop this therapy if it does not help me?
How much will this therapy cost?
How will this therapy burden my family (either financially or physically) if a prolonged recovery time is required?

Can a person who has dementia, mental retardation, or mental illness give informed consent?

Any person who can understand the nature of his or her disease, appreciate his or her options for treatment, and make a voluntary, unconstrained choice is capable of giving a legally valid informed consent or refusal. Further, any person with any of these conditions who is able to give informed consent is also able to prepare an advance directive. A person's capacity to give informed consent may vary over time, however, so that today someone may be unable to understand or freely choose, while tomorrow that person may be able to do so. An example of such a circumstance is the patient with early Alzheimer's disease, whose ability to give informed consent can vary from day to day or even hour to hour. In our experience, many mentally ill and retarded individuals, as well as those with early dementia, have been able to consent to an advance directive.

Can minors give informed consent?

To a certain extent, yes. As children grow up, they mature in both physical and intellectual ways. A boy at sevven may be able to contribute his perceptions of whether he wants to be treated for an illness, although his parents will ultimately be responsible for giving informed consent. As the child matures through adolescence, the capacity to reason, weigh alternatives, and make choices generally increases. Hence, the same boy at seventeen may be able to give informed consent, if his state laws permit it.

Current laws governing the execution of living wills and durable powers of attorney exclude minors. Although minors of a certain age (the age differs by state) cannot sign a binding power of attorney or living will, they *can* express their wishes about life-sustaining medical therapies, by discussing the issues with their parents and their doctor.

Why should informed consent be important to me?

The physician's duty to solicit an informed consent guarantees your ability to make your own choices and expect that they will be honored. Although physicians may know more about your condition and your treatment options than you do, you have the right to be given enough information to make your own decisions about medical treatments. The physician's responsibility to ensure an informed consent thereby offsets the possibility of paternalistic coercion that could force a particular decision in the informed consent process.

Informed choices are supported by the principle of autonomy, which grounds the patient's right to decide freely when to continue medical treatments and when to discontinue nonbeneficial treatments. This guarantees your decision-making capability within the medical care system as well as your doctor's responsibility to honor your choices. Regardless of how strongly a physician may feel about his or her obligation to make you better again, you have a right to say no to medical treatment. However, the physician has professional autonomy.

What does the physician's professional autonomy have to do with me?

Physicians have the right not to be forced to violate their own moral, professional, or religious codes, provided they do not abandon a patient. If you go to a doctor who has strong views that conflict with your choices, he or she has a right to withdraw from your care, as long as responsibility for your care is transferred to another doctor (this right is recognized in most advance directive legislation). All of us, including physicians, have values that underlie our attitudes and influence our behaviors.

What is justice?

Justice is the principle of dealing fairly and equitably with people. Sometimes, in the context of medicine, justice is interpreted as being related to the allocation of limited resources. Broadly interpreted, however, justice encompasses fair and equitable treatment of persons under whatever system is being considered.

How is justice important in medicine?

Justice has become increasingly important in medicine as the money available for health care seems to become increasingly insufficient to meet people's medical needs. As a result, constraints have been placed on hospitals which are intended to curb the amount of money spent on health care. Decisions about length of hospital stays for procedures and administration of medical therapies are increasingly being regulated by the U.S. government. The government implemented these programs to help distribute funds to hospitals more fairly, so that monies are allocated more equitably to provide for the health care needs of more people.

Can justice interfere with other principles?

Justice-based concerns of trying to share the cost of health care more equitably could interfere with other principles if these considerations influenced the physician's or hospital's decision to hospitalize a patient.

Treatment decisions based solely on economic considerations—rather than on the patient's benefit— would be ethically suspect. On the other hand, sometimes "high-tech," high-cost therapies are not medically justifiable. For instance, every time you get a headache, your doctor shouldn't request a computer-enhanced scan of the brain (and neither should you). To do so would enormously drive up the costs of medical care for everyone.

Where do I fit into this picture?

As a patient, you have certain rights that must be respected within the health care field. You have the right to receive sound medical therapy and the right to refuse that therapy. Further, you have the right to expect that no one will coerce individual medical practitioners or health care facilities into changing the practice of medicine in a way that would adversely affect the delivery of health care. You fit in as a consumer safeguarding your own interests within the system.

4

The Value of Values

What are values?

Values are the beliefs we hold that allow us to frame our perspective of life from day to day. They can be religious, cultural, or philosophical in nature. Values develop as we grow up within our families, our communities, and society.

Why are values important?

Values are important because they help to formulate the decisions we may make in our lives. The values we hold help guide our opinions of the world around us and help us make decisions about our place in that world. By examining our own values, we can better understand *how* we perceive the world and *why* we perceive it as we do.

What are attitudes?

Attitudes describe the feeling we have about the things we encounter in life. Attitudes are based on our emotional and intellectual reactions and reflections. Positive or negative attitudes toward challenges, setbacks, and success, for example, are part of the value system we have developed. We develop these attitudes in response to our experiences with the world. The projection of our attitudes to others in part reflects the values that we hold.

How do values and attitudes interact?

Values and attitudes interact by reflecting the nature of one another. Our values help to form the attitudes we project to others. If we hold values that reflect a certain belief system, our attitudes will likely also reflect those values outwards, to others. The interaction between our values and our attitudes is often not even recognized by us, however.

What are behaviors?

Behaviors are the methods we use to demonstrate our values and attitudes. Behaviors come in the form of action and in the form of inaction. The way in which we conduct ourselves in the world and with those around us—this is our behavior.

How do values and attitudes affect behaviors?

Values and attitudes act as a catalyst for the way we behave toward others. For example, if we hold values and attitudes that are critical of a particular action, it is likely that our behavior will reflect this: we probably will not engage in that action. Likewise, if our values and attitudes include a belief that it is worthwhile to do a particular thing, our behavior will probably reflect that fact. We do not always behave in accord with our attitudes, however. Sometimes we engage in actions that do not necessarily "fit in" with the attitudes we project (for example, a conservative, practical person may impulsively buy a sports car).

Are medical values different from other values?

Medical values are similar to the other values that we hold throughout life. Medical values, though, are directed toward a specific part of life: the medical world. For example, we may broadly value being free as individuals; a corresponding medical value would address our wish to have freedom and respect shown to us when we make medical decisions for ourselves.

How can medical values play a role in my attitudes and behaviors?

Your values will be reflected in your attitudes, and these, in turn, will direct your behavior. For example, if you value being informed about your medical care to improve your health, and if you value your freedom to choose medical therapies, these values will be reflected in the attitudes you have toward health care. Along with your reflections on past personal experiences, these attitudes will contribute to your behavior concerning health care decisions as well as to how you behave when you interact with your doctor.

Are medical values related to advance directives?

Recent research conducted by Dr. David Doukas and Dr. Daniel Gorenflo has revealed that certain medical values do appear to be related to the formulation of advance directives. In two recent investigations, the selection of values and advance directives was studied in two different populations: a multi-generational population and an outpatient population of well adults.

Participants in these studies were asked to rank their agreement with a variety of important values in medical care as well as the desirability of several medical therapies listed in the Values History (see the Appendix). In both studies, patient values based on imposing burdens on the family were inversely correlated with the preferences toward life-sustaining medical therapies for terminal illness. In other words, the more intense the person's concern about family burden, the less likely the person was to want life-sustaining medical therapies. (Family burden values included items such as being a financial or physical burden on other members of the family.) Medical values regarding having wishes carried out by a physician were not shown to be relevant to advance directive preferences in these populations. These findings may reflect a pragmatic concern by the patient about pain- and burden-related issues. These findings may also suggest that participants lacked knowledge about patient rights involved in medical decision making.

Should I discuss my values with my family?

Yes. Discussing your values with your family allows them to understand the medical values you hold. Your family will better understand your medical decisions and will likely be more accepting should these preferences need to be carried out. These discussions allow for an open exchange of ideas between you and your family, so there is no chance for a misunderstanding about why you wish to sign an advance directive.

When a family member acts as a proxy for another person, there is a presumption that the family member has an intimate knowledge of the patient's values and preferences, or is at least trusted enough to be named as proxy in a durable power of attorney for health care. Such knowledge is based on a relationship of trust and understanding, in which values and medical preferences are discussed. If such discussions do not take place, the patient may someday be done a grave disservice. (For information about the various values that can be discussed, see chapter 6.)

Is there anyone else with whom I ought to consider discussing my values?

You should have discussions with the person you are likely to select as your proxy. This person may or may not be a family member. It may be quite helpful for you to discuss your values regarding medical care with your religious or spiritual adviser, who can help you clarify or better articulate your religious and philosophical values. Such discussions are intended to help you discover your own values, though, rather than to allow someone else to tell you what values you should believe in. This process is introspective and reflective—the answers come from within you.

Will my doctor find it helpful to be acquainted with my values?

Yes. Information about your values will give your doctor insight into the factors that contributed to your decision to sign an advance directive. By knowing about the values and attitudes you hold, your doctor may better understand your decisions.

It is impossible to imagine all the many scenarios of illness, or to predict which illnesses any of us will encounter (including in what way we might become terminally ill or otherwise unable to recover), but we can communicate our *general* medical values and attitudes to others, and this information may prove very helpful to them. If you have discussed these ideas with your family and your doctor, and then someday you're unable to talk for yourself or express yourself, your doctor will be able, with the assistance of your family, to interpret your preferences on medical treatment in a broader light.

Why will I find it helpful to explore my own values?

Thinking about these values now can help you prepare to make future decisions. People tend to put off thinking about advance directives, but since, as we've said, it's impossible to predict when a life-threatening illness or accident might occur, we recommend that, if you haven't already done so, you start thinking about your medical values now. Then you may have a better understanding of why signing an advance directive might be an important action for you to take.

Will my values change over time?

It is very likely that your values will change over your lifetime. We are all dynamic creatures, and as we experience new positive and negative events, our values change. How much they change—whether just slightly or dramatically—depends upon how firmly we believe in our value system when we encounter such events. As a result, it is wise to update any method of values assessment periodically (we recommend doing this every six to twelve months). This allows you to reflect on the latest events in your life and to examine what effect they have had on your value system.

When should I discuss my values with others?

There is no "best time" to discuss your values with either your family or your doctor; nor is there any good reason to delay doing so. Given the unpredictability of life, we advise you to discuss your values with your family and doctor as soon as possible, so that other people will be familiar with your medical values should you become unable to make decisions. Communicating these values is particularly helpful when communication is accompanied by a written decision concerning what you would want done under certain circumstances. As stated repeatedly throughout this book, beginning in the Preface, this decision can be formalized using a living will, a durable power of attorney for health care, or a Values History. We turn to the first two of these advance directives in the next chapter.

5

The Living Will and the Durable Power of Attorney for Health Care

Why were advance directives developed?

Advance directives were first developed to allow people to tell their doctors and family what kinds of medical therapies they wish to refuse in case of terminal illness. As technology has advanced over the years and has become better able to keep people alive longer, many people have wanted a method to say "enough is enough." Indeed, some people have voiced the fear that they will somehow be sustained on medical machines and therapies against their will.

Competent people have the right to consent to or refuse any medical therapy that could benefit them. Advance directives provide a way for a person to state in advance which medical treatments are desired and which are not desired under certain circumstances, and then have these wishes carried out if he or she later is unable to make or express a choice when a health care decision must be made.

When were advance directives developed?

Living wills were developed in the mid-1970s, beginning with the 1976 Natural Death Act in California and eventually spreading across forty-seven states and the District of Columbia.

The durable power of attorney for health care, which allows for the appointment of a surrogate decision maker for health care (also called an *agent,* or *proxy*), was developed more recently. Durable powers of attorney for health care have been legalized explicitly by statute in most states, while durable powers of attorney can be used in all states.

What is the purpose of these advance directives?

Both living wills and durable powers of attorney for health care allow a person to express health care preferences that are to be implemented in a future circumstance of incapacity. The foundation of a person's ability to sign a living will or durable power of attorney is informed consent. As discussed in chapter 3, informed consent is the autonomous right of the person to approve or refuse a medical therapy or plan that has been offered or recommended to him or her. As noted, three phases— disclosure, comprehension, and freedom from constraint—comprise informed consent.

What is a terminal illness?

A terminal illness is generally understood to be an illness that will inevitably lead to death, despite medical intervention. Medical intervention may prolong the life of the person, but the disease process continues. As we have explained elsewhere in this book, medical intervention may be said to prolong dying in some cases.

How is persistent vegetative state defined?

A persistently vegetative state is an irreversible neurological condition in which a person can no longer respond knowingly to others or communicate with them in any way but is capable of breathing on his or her own. A person in a persistently vegetative state has suffered damage to the brain as a result of a lack of oxygen. This damage impairs the person's ability to think, feel, reason, and communicate. A person in a persistently vegetative state may exhibit reflex responses to certain stimuli and may go through what appear to be sleep and wake cycles, but the person will not be able to perceive what is going on around him or her and will not be able to communicate with others.

A persistently vegetative state is different from an irreversible coma. A person in an irreversible coma is permanently in a sleep-like state and has no wakeful episodes. The person is not able to communicate and does not have sleep-wake cycles. An irreversible coma is the result of irreparable damage to massive areas of the brain caused by oxygen deprivation.

A reversible coma is usually the result of acute, but less severe, injury to the brain from trauma (an automobile accident, for example) or from a drug overdose. The person will eventually "come out" of this kind of coma.

What is incapacity?

In the context of the topic of this book, incapacity means an inability to understand the treatment choices presented, to appreciate the implications of the available alternatives, and to make and communicate a decision about health care.

Decision-making capacity is sometimes (though not always) defined in state laws governing health care decisions and advance directives. Usually, before an advance directive becomes operational, one or two physicians must examine the person and certify that he or she lacks the capacity to make a decision.

How is incapacity related to advance directives?

You have the right to make your own health care decisions as long as you possess the decision-making capacity to do so. Whether or not you have signed a living will or a durable power of attorney for health care, when you have the capacity to make decisions (or if you lose that capacity but later regain it), you have the right to make these decisions yourself.

It is only when you lose your decision-making capacity that advance directives may become critical in your health care. If you become incapacitated and are unable to make health care decisions, then an advance directive can speak in your place. On the other hand, if you become incapacitated and do not have an advance directive, your family and your doctor may be forced into trying to make a decision for you, based on your general attitudes and values. Under some circumstances, a court may have to make decisions for you or authorize a family member or friend to do so. Making medical decisions for an incapacitated person based on his or her formal expression of medical values and preferences in an advance directive is far easier than making these same decisions based on general impressions of that person's life values.

Who can sign an advance directive?

Any adult person who has the capacity to formulate an informed consent can sign an advance directive.

An advance directive may not be applicable under certain conditions, however. Some states limit the right of pregnant patients to refuse certain treatments, for example, in order to protect the developing fetus.

What might motivate me to sign a living will or a durable power of attorney for health care?

An individual's motivation for signing a living will or a durable power of attorney for health care is based upon the desire (and the right) to decide what sort of therapies he or she would want and not want if he or she were ever unable to voice a consent or refusal. Further, these documents allow the person who has a known illness to declare which therapies in his or her current medical condition would be acceptable and which should not be started or continued in future circumstances, should the illness lead to decision-making incapacity. They give the person the opportunity to voice personal values and goals in a well-reasoned statement that allows the physician to understand the person's rationale for choosing to accept or refuse such care. Not making such a declaration may jeopardize your ability to be treated in the manner of your choosing if you should someday be unable to speak for yourself.

With the passage of the Patient Self-Determination Act, patients will be given more opportunities than in the past to learn about advance directives. The problem with the Act lies in the circumstances under which it is carried out. That is, unless you are enrolled in a health maintenance organization, the forms will probably not be given to you (unless you obtain them on your own) until you are admitted to a hospital, nursing home, hospice, or other health agency. That may be too late, however, because you may not be able to fill out an advance directive at that time—you may be unconscious, or you may be in too much pain. You may one day put your loved ones in the difficult position of selecting therapies for you based on their guesses about what you would choose. Also, if you don't have an advance directive and you someday become unable to communicate, you may be subjected to medical therapies that you do not want. We urge you to sign an advance directive *now*, while you are thinking about your values for medical care.

Whom should I choose as my proxy or agent for my durable power of attorney for health care?

You can select any adult who you think would best represent your values and preferences regarding medical therapies. This person should be well acquainted with your values and preferences. While many people choose a relative to serve as their proxy, a proxy can be anyone (a spouse, a friend, a significant other) who can accurately convey your wishes to a health care team if you are unable to speak for yourself.

Before you sign a durable power of attorney which specifies the person who will serve as your agent, you must ask that person whether he or she is willing to do so, since the proxy assumes a serious responsibility on agreeing to convey your instructions to your doctor. The proxy designate can be assured that you will not be charging him or her with making decisions based on his or her own personal judgment and values, however. Rather, the proxy is responsible for serving as a conduit between you and your doctor. Such reassurance makes it clear to a prospective proxy that the decisions are actually coming from you (through your stated or recorded values and preferences), and not from the proxy.

It is also important to impress on your proxy the desirability of reviewing your health care values and preferences on a periodic basis, so that he or she is kept updated. You can take the initiative to see that this happens. Also, your proxy should be reassured that he or she is not financially responsible for your care on the basis of this designation alone.

Can my doctor serve as my proxy?

No. Your doctor cannot serve as your proxy because of the conflict of interest that may arise between the physician's role of healing and the fulfillment of the patient's autonomous preferences. Also, in many states your doctor is prohibited by law from serving as your proxy.

Are the forms for living wills and durable powers of attorney for health care the same in all states?

Not exactly. There are differences in the way state legislatures have written some of the statutes. These differences may affect both the form and the content of advance directives. You must learn about *your own state's laws* regarding the living will and the durable power of attorney in order to understand how the documents are used in your state.

Common features of durable powers of attorney for health care are: identification of the person (or persons) appointed to act as your agent (or agents) if you are incapacitated; the ability to apply this empowerment to all medical decision making on your behalf; and the ability to provide detailed instructions that you want your agent to follow if you are unable to speak for yourself.

Common features of living will statutes are: the right to include personalized instructions; the need for one or two physicians to certify that the patient is terminally ill prior to implementation; the requirement of the doctor either to follow the provisions of a valid living will or to transfer care of the patient; the requirement of the doctor to incorporate a known living will into the medical record; the requirement to have two witnesses to the patient's signing of the document; and a release of the doctor and health facility from liability for following the living will.

Some states have passed living will statutes that do not allow for the withdrawal or withholding of nutrition and hydration (although some state courts have declared that limitation unconstitutional). In other states, living wills are not effective if the patient is pregnant. Some states allow for family consent or oral declarations of a living will (nevertheless, we recommend that everyone provide a *written* statement, which permits portability and verification). Many living will laws require doctors who cannot carry out the living will to transfer the patient to another doctor who will honor it. Some states explicitly allow for the honoring of a living will signed in another state, while others do not address that issue. (Patients who live part-time in two or more states may want to sign a declaration that is valid for both states or, conversely, sign living wills that are valid in each of the states.)

Your own state's versions of the durable power of attorney for health care and the living will are likely to be worded slightly differently from other states' and will cover different aspects of health care. That's why it's best to obtain a copy of your own state's advance directives. (If your state has not yet passed an advance directive by statute, you can use a generic living will or durable power of attorney, as provided in the Appendix.)

Despite minor differences, the forms are so similar between states that a document executed in one state is likely to be honored in another state, to the extent permitted under local laws. But, again, to be safe, it's best to obtain a document that has been approved for use in *your* state. (Instructions for obtaining these forms are provided in chapter 8 and the Appendix.)

Do I have to consult anyone before I sign?

No, there is no requirement that you consult with anyone before you sign an advance directive. Nevertheless, we believe you should review your values, attitudes, and preferences with your physician before you sign an advance directive, so that you're certain you have an adequate understanding of the consequences of your decisions.

Through such a discussion, you *and your doctor* will gain a much better understanding of what you are consenting to or refusing, and why. In this way, you will be making informed choices, rather than independently signing an advance directive without having the benefit of adequate knowledge and reflection. At the same time, your doctor will better understand your motivations for making the decisions you make, and for signing an advance directive in the first place. (Chapters 6 and 8 explain how to sign an advance directive.)

Is there a possibility that my doctor won't know enough about advance directives to help me?

It is possible, but unlikely. Recent research indicates that physicians know a great deal about advance directives, but that physicians can benefit from having more information about them and more experience with their use. It also appears that physicians too often wait for patients to bring the subject up.

National studies have not yet been conducted on the durable power of attorney for health care, but research has been done recently on the living will. In a nationwide survey, Dr. Doukas and his colleagues asked more than four hundred family physicians about their knowledge of, clinical use of, and personal use of the living will.* Information about physician-initiated and patient-

*D. J. Doukas, D. W. Gorenflo, and S. S. Coughlin, "The Living Will: A National Survey," *Family Medicine*, 1991, 23(5):354–56.

initiated discussions of the living will was also elicited. Physicians were asked to give their view as to the appropriateness of the living will and to identify their sources of information about the living will.

Of the respondents, 95 percent reported being aware of the living will, while 69 percent reported using the living will clinically (that is, they have used living wills in caring for patients). Only 51 percent of the physicians responding reported that they initiated discussions with their patients, while 71 percent of the physicians reported that their patients had come to them to initiate conversations about the living will. Those physicians who knew the most about the living will also were most likely to use the living will clinically, to initiate discussion with patients, to perceive the living will as useful, and to sign the document themselves. Notably, about 25 percent of the physicians who reported not initiating discussions with patients gave lack of knowledge as the reason. In other words, the more doctors know about living wills, the more they seem to value and use them, both professionally and personally.

When asked how they had learned of the living will, 56 percent of the physicians cited their patients; 47 percent, the medical literature; and 31 percent, the media. It appears that patients have more influence on doctors than we realize! When asked when it is appropriate to discuss the subject of the living will, 74 percent of the physicians said they consider it appropriate with a patient who is debilitated and has a poor prognosis; 62 percent, with any HIV-infected patient; and 58 percent, with any elderly patient. Twelve percent of physicians agreed with the statement that "the initiative should always come from the patient."

This nationwide survey revealed three factors that may distinguish between use and non-use of the living will: physician knowledge, physician initiation of discussion, and physician appraisal of the appropriateness of the living will based on the severity of the patient's illness. Studies such as this one help physicians gain a better understanding of what motivates them to offer the living will and other advance directives to their patients. It also demonstrates the necessity for patients to be more demanding of their physicians when it comes to a discussion of advance directives.

Do I need witnesses when I sign an advance directive?

Yes. On the advance directive forms you will find a description of the intent of the form: to stipulate that you will forgo treatment if terminally ill (on the living will) and that you transfer decision-making authority to a proxy if incapacitated (on the durable power of attorney for health care). Below this description are lines for your signature and the date, and lines for witnesses to sign at the same time. For both the living will and the durable power of attorney for health care, witnesses must sign the document at the same time you do.

Why are witnesses required?

To show that the person who signed did so knowingly and freely. The signatures of witnesses show that you actually signed the directive, and they may also serve as testimonials to your competence at the time of the signing. Under these circumstances the document is far less likely to be challenged in the future (again, this depends on state law).

Can anyone serve as a witness?

A witness should not be a relative, a health care provider, an employee of a health care provider, or an heir of the person whose directive is being formalized. These provisions guard against any possible conflict of interest.

Why is soundness of mind necessary when I sign an advance directive?

Soundness of mind is necessary because you must understand the importance and implications of an advance directive in order for it to be valid. The voluntary nature of the decision to execute an advance directive helps to guarantee that you were not coerced to make the decision, that your decision was not made in a frivolous manner, and that you were not in a mentally unbalanced state when you made the decision.

How long are advance directives valid?

Several state statutes originally required that living wills be renewed periodically. Now, all states that allow a living will by statute have revised of those laws, so that once a living will is signed, it remains valid unless the patient revokes it. Durable powers of attorney for health care also last indefinitely, unless the person writing the document decides to limit the time during which it will be effective.

What happens if I want to withdraw or change my advance directive?

You can revoke a living will or durable power of attorney for health care by destroying it or by writing the word *void* across it. You always have the right to revoke a living will. Revoking a living will means that you *do want life-sustaining therapies* begun or continued if you are terminally ill or persistently vegetative. You can also change the person to whom you give decision-making authority, or modify your specific instructions about health care. You can execute a new advance directive and make it clear that this document supersedes all previously executed directives. Signing an advance directive today does not mean that you can't change your mind later. You *can*.

6

The Values History: Defining Your Health Care Values

What is the Values History?

The Values History, developed by Dr. David Doukas and Dr. Laurence McCullough, is an instrument designed to enhance current advance directives.* (The term *value history* was coined by Dr. Edmund Pellegrino in the early 1980s to describe the discussions that might take place that would enable a doctor to elicit the values that are important to a patient's health care decisions.) The Values History by Doukas and McCullough is intended to supplement a living will or durable power of attorney by

---

*D. Doukas and L. McCullough, "The Values History: The Evaluation of the Patient's Values and Advance Directives," *Journal of Family Practice*, February 1991, 32(1): 145–53; D. Doukas, S. Lipson, and L. McCullough, "Value History," in *Clinical Aspects of Aging*, 3d ed., ed. W. Reichel (Baltimore: Williams and Wilkins, 1989): 615–16; D. Doukas and L. McCullough, "Truth Telling and Confidentiality in the Aged Patient," ibid., 609–15; D. Doukas and L. McCullough, "Assessing the Values History of the Aged Patient Regarding Critical and Chronic Care," in *Handbook of Geriatric Assessment*, ed. J. Gallo, W. Reichel, and L. Andersen (Rockville, Md.: Aspen Press, 1988): 111–24.

stimulating a person's thinking about specific medical values and eliciting from people statements concerning the values that would be important to them in the event of a terminal illness or if they were in a persistently vegetative state. Further, the Values History contains explicit advance directive statements regarding many medical therapies. An individual can complete these statements and be assured that the document will clearly state his or her wishes to family members and health care personnel. (The Values History is reproduced in the Appendix.)

This document allows the person to specify for each therapy the person's acceptance or rejection of that therapy or—a third alternative—the person's willingness to permit the health care team to attempt a trial of intervention for that therapy. In a *trial of intervention*, a therapy is carried out for a specified period or as long as it takes to determine either that a specific benefit will be gained through the therapy or that the therapy is futile.

The Values History has been shown to be a valuable contribution to the advance directive process. Other, similarly named, attempts either have focused entirely on the directive aspect of decision making (without asking the patient about values) or have asked open-ended, global questions about patient values. While these efforts are helpful additions to the advance directive literature, we believe that using the Values History by Doukas and McCullough has the following advantage: by allowing you to reflect *meaningfully* on your *medical values* and by preparing you to formulate *specific* advance directives, the Values History allows you to express your values more meaningfully and more specifically than other documents do. At the same time, the Values History facilitates your reflection on these important values through a series of questions and statements.

What kinds of questions does the Values History ask?

The Values History helps you express your values by, first, inquiring which is more important to you at the end of your life: a good quality of life, regardless of whether that life is shortened, or a longer length of life, regardless of the quality of that life. This choice is fundamental in terms of medical values.

The Values History next lists many values having to do with such issues as your ability to communicate, your desire to have your doctor carry out your wishes, and your wish to avoid placing various burdens on your family due to your illness. The Values History asks you to circle those values that are most meaningful to you. You are also encouraged to add other values that are important to you, and to expand on your previously voiced values.

Finally, the Values History turns to a series of medical interventions that are possible and assesses your preferences regarding these interventions. Both acute interventions (such as cardiopulmonary resuscitation and ventilator use) and chronic interventions (such as feeding tube use and dialysis) are considered in the Values History. We think it is crucial for you and your doctor to discuss these therapies and how they might be important for you. (Chapter 8 describes the steps involved in completing the Values History.)

Are there legal barriers to use of the Values History?

The Values History is an important asset in the informed consent or refusal process for both ethical and legal reasons. It has standing ethically under the right of any competent adult to make an informed and free medical treatment decision. It also has legal standing to the extent that states allow you to add specific instructions to your living will and durable power of attorney. It is intended that the Values History be attached as an addendum to a valid signed living will or durable power of attorney for health care.

A few states currently limit some of the types of decisions you might make (such as refusing nutrition and hydration) in your Values History, but you should state preferences anyway. Perhaps the laws will change in the future. It is also possible that you will be in a different jurisdiction when a decision must be made about your care.

It is always helpful for others to understand your values and preferences, especially if they are being asked to make decisions for you.

Besides legal barriers, is there anything else that might obstruct the implementation of my preferences in my Values History?

Sometimes doctors and family members attempt to interfere with the implementation of a person's preferences as stated in an advance directive. If your doctor is not willing to carry out your advance directives, he or she should promptly arrange to transfer your care to another doctor. If your family or friends feel that your doctor is not carrying out your wishes, they ought to arrange for your care to be transferred.

When a family tries to obstruct fulfillment of your advance directives, it is usually because of a conflict of intent (resulting in overtreatment due to "caring") or conflict of interest (this is discussed further in chapter 7). Sometimes it is difficult to know how you would view a particular medical condition; different people may disagree on how to interpret or apply your Values History. If this happens, then the doctor and family members may seek the advice and counsel of an ethics committee.

How can the Values History help me?

The Values History can be helpful to you if you have strong feelings about protecting yourself from pain or protecting your family against harm or burden, if you have concerns about voicing your health care decisions, and if you have preferences about how you want your physician to comply with your desires. By listing these values, you can clarify for the health care team the values that underlie the advance directives you select.

The articulation of your medical values may be of great benefit to those who may, in the future, need to interpret the intent of your previously signed advance directives. By clearly stating your medical values and directives regarding treatment, you enable others to carry out your wishes by allowing for the broader interpretation of your values and directives in future, unforeseen medical circumstances. No one can predict what medical situation may someday threaten his or her life, and no living will or durable power of attorney can cover all medical contingencies. The Values History is intended to supplement a living will or durable power of attorney for health care that you have already signed. The Values History gives these documents fuller meaning, so that unforeseen events can be addressed with the guidance of your medical values and directives.

How does the Values History help me discuss my treatment preferences and values with my doctor and family?

Physicians and families can act as sounding boards, helping you think through decisions on advance directives. The Values History encourages you to hold these discussions, in that it asks questions about your own individual values. The questioning and answering that goes on between you and your physician, and you and your family, increases your capacity to understand your own feelings, values, and attitudes as well as the implications of your treatment decisions. As we have discussed, all of these influence the formulation of a living will or a durable power of attorney.

The discussions you have now and in the future with your doctor may one day be very important for your health care. These discussions will help your doctor understand the circumstances of illness under which you would want your advance directives carried out. Holding these discussions frankly and openly helps avoid misunderstandings about your wishes regarding life-sustaining therapy.

Do I have only two options? Must I either agree to a treatment or refuse it?

Your advance directives regarding health care need not be absolute. In the Values History, you are free to voice your preferences to specific directives in a method of *limited consent* known as a *trial of intervention*. A trial of intervention allows you to designate a length of time after which you would want a therapy stopped or a circumstance under which you would want a therapy stopped.

In a trial of intervention, a therapy is initiated and then monitored to determine whether it will be of benefit. If the therapy doesn't help after a *time period that you set*, it can be discontinued. For example, if you designate a trial of intervention to allow the use of a ventilator for two weeks and if the ventilator proves to be nonbeneficial during this time, and recovery is deemed hopeless, your doctor could then honor your wish to discontinue its use. Conversely, you could designate a trial of intervention whereby the therapy is continued, *provided that it is medically beneficial* to you (regardless of the duration of the intervention). If the therapy is initiated and, after a period considered reasonable by the physician and by you or your proxy, it renders you no benefit, the therapy would be discontinued.

It is important to discuss these options with your doctor. In particular, a decision to consent to a trial of intervention without a definitive time limit needs to be based on a great deal of trust between you and your doctor. For example, let us imagine two patients with known chronic kidney disease, both of whom wish to describe to their doctor the terms of their trial of intervention to continue on dialysis. One patient desires a four-week trial of intervention of dialysis if a terminal illness or persistent vegetative state is present, and stipulates that if progress toward ameliorating the disease is not evident at two weeks, the therapy would be discontinued. The other patient, given the same circumstances, desires a trial based on the presence of medical benefit, stipulating that if no progress is being made in treatment of the condition, the therapy would be discontinued (regardless of the timing). The latter option is more open-ended but allows for implementation based on the absence or presence of medical benefit, which may become medically evident before a set time interval has elapsed.

It is important to remember that a doctor is not *required* to initiate or continue a therapy just because you have agreed to have that therapy. As discussed in chapter 2, if your condition is such that use of the therapy would be futile, there is no obligation on the part of the doctor to use it. When a person selects trial of intervention, that person is conveying his values and preferences regarding the use of that therapy more accurately than he or she would by simply saying "yes" to it.

Why does the Values History ask me *why* I have made the decision I have made?

After your consent or refusal to each intervention, the Values History asks you why you have made this choice. This question gives you an opportunity to articulate the reasons, values, or experiences that influenced your decision. This information may be valuable to your doctor and family if such interventions are being considered when you are unable to speak for yourself.

In the next several pages we describe the various acute and chronic medical interventions included in the Directives Section of the Values History, in their order of presentation (the document itself appears in the Appendix). Reviewing what's involved in the use of these therapies will help you decide how you wish to respond to these items in the Values History. In addition to reading about these therapies here, you should discuss them with your doctor. It is important that you understand these therapies and the possible outcomes of their use before you complete the Values History (see chapter 8 for instructions on how to complete the document).

What is CPR?

Cardiopulmonary resuscitation, or CPR, refers to a broad spectrum of medical interventions that are employed to "restart" a person's heart or lungs after they have stopped working (that is, when they are said to be in a state of "arrest"). The methods used in CPR to attempt to restore bodily function include the manual compression of the chest, accomplished by pressing vigorously on the chest with both hands, and electro-cardioversion (or electrical shocking of the chest), both of which are performed in an attempt to restart the heart, as well as introduction of air into the lungs by means of a mask over the mouth and nose or by means of an endotracheal tube (which allows oxygen to be delivered directly into the lungs). Cardiopulmonary resuscitation may also take the form of an injection of any of a vast array of cardiac medications that are used to attempt to restore normal electrical conduction within the heart after an arrest has occurred.

It should be noted that CPR efforts, performed with the intent of benefiting the patient, may carry unwanted or undesirable burdens. These efforts may result in rib fractures, electrical burns of the patient's chest, or a pneumothorax (the introduction of air between the lungs and the chest wall). An endotracheal tube may cause pain when introduced into the patient's respiratory system to control breathing during this emergency. CPR may be carried out with the intention of benefiting the patient, but there is potential for discomfort as a result of such efforts.

What is a ventilator?

A ventilator (also called a respirator) is a mechanical device that provides artificial respiration (breathing) by the person's lungs when the person is unable to breathe on his or her own. A ventilator controls the number of breaths the person takes each minute, the volume of breaths, and the percentage of oxygen in each breath. A ventilator permits the doctor to maintain precise control over the breathing of the patient. A ventilator can be put in place either through a tracheostomy (the surgical insertion of a tube through the neck into the windpipe) or through an endotracheal tube.

What is an endotracheal tube?

An endotracheal tube is a clear plastic tube that is inserted into the mouth and down the throat by way of the vocal cords to the trachea. It allows for the free passage of air between the mouth and the lungs. The endotracheal tube is used to ensure that a patient's airway remains open when cardiopulmonary resuscitation is performed or a ventilator is used. (Long-term use of a ventilator usually requires the surgical procedure, the tracheostomy.) The endotracheal tube is an intervention that many people, particularly people with chronic lung disease, have negative feelings about, based on past personal or family experiences.

What are nasogastric tubes, gastrostomy tubes, and other enteral feeding tubes, and how do they relate to nutrition and hydration?

A feeding tube delivers food to a person when the person no longer is able to eat by mouth or when it is not medically safe for the person to eat by mouth. The food is processed so that it is easily delivered to the person through the tube. Feeding tubes are medically indicated when there is a good chance that food delivered by mouth will be accidentally aspirated (diverted) into the lungs, resulting in pneumonia.

A nasogastric tube is a feeding tube that is placed through the nose, down the esophagus, and into the stomach. (The esophagus is the body's connection between the mouth and the stomach.) A gastrostomy tube is placed into the stomach or small intestine through a hole surgically opened in the side of the abdomen. Such tubes may also be referred to, less specifically, as enteral feeding tubes, since they can also deliver food into the small intestine (*enteral* means *intestinal*). An enteral feeding tube is usually used when it is anticipated that the patient will not regain the ability to eat by mouth.

What is total parenteral nutrition?

Total parenteral nutrition, also known as TPN, is a method of providing nutritional substances directly into the bloodstream through the veins. The tubes can be inserted through the large central veins or through smaller peripheral veins. TPN is generally used when a patient is unable to eat for a prolonged period and has difficulty digesting food. TPN is particularly beneficial for temporary use after an operation has been performed on the gastrointestinal tract. Because nutrition is provided straight into the bloodstream, entirely bypassing the stomach and bowels, these organs have a chance to rest and to heal. When someone is unable to process food in the gastrointestinal tract for a longer duration, however, it may be necessary to use TPN for a sustained period of time.

What do intravenous medication and intravenous hydration mean?

Intravenous medication means having medicines administered by vein; intravenous hydration means having solutions administered by vein to provide your body with necessary fluids and chemicals to sustain life. A directive concerning these two interventions would be operative in such diverse settings as hospital, home care, hospice, and long-term care.

Should you become terminally ill or enter a persistently vegetative state, medicines intended to treat your illness would not be administered intravenously if you state beforehand that you consider such efforts to be fruitless under those circumstances. On the other hand, medicines necessary for the control of pain *would* be administered, and other comfort care measures *would* be provided, should you become terminally ill or be in a persistently vegetative state. Similarly, life-sustaining fluids would not be administered if you state beforehand that receiving such fluids would not be acceptable to you if you were dying or if you were permanently unable to wake up.

What does it mean to consider the use of all medications used for the treatment of my illness?

This language refines the intent of the previous directive to specify consent to or refusal of all methods of treatment delivery. With a treatment refusal to this directive, oral medications, subcutaneous medications (injected under the skin), or injections of medications into the muscle would not be used in the circumstances of terminal illness or persistently vegetative state. *With all medication refusal directives, the use of pain medication to alleviate suffering is permitted.*

What is dialysis?

Dialysis is a process whereby the blood is filtered through a machine that removes waste from the blood when the kidneys can no longer perform this function. Dialysis may be needed acutely—temporarily—in response to acute kidney failure (such as kidney failure caused by infection or immune system disorders), or it may be performed indefinitely, if, for example, a chronic disease has caused a person's kidneys to fail.

What is an autopsy?

An autopsy is a procedure wherein a body is examined after death to find out what led to death. The reason for a person's death is often unclear, but by examining the body's organs, the medical team can usually determine what the cause of death was.

We recommend that you consent to an autopsy in an advance directive, because autopsy results are helpful. An autopsy provides the family with useful information, particularly if the disease that caused death is one that may afflict other family members. Autopsies help the medical team better understand the nature of the disease that caused death and will advance understanding of the disease. Thus, an investigation into the cause of your death may be helpful to others. Be assured that after autopsy, your body will be returned to your family for any desired religious services and burial that you or they request. Autopsy is not disfiguring to the portions of the body that would be visible if you or your family wish to have an open-casket service.

In some states, autopsies may not be carried out without your family's consent except when required by statute or court order. By clearly stating your wishes regarding autopsy in an advance directive, you may help your family decide to respect your wish for an autopsy and to provide the necessary consent.

What is organ donation?

Organ donation allows you to make a gift of your organs or other tissues (for example, your heart, liver, or corneas, or grafts from your skin) to others after you have been declared dead by your doctor. All fifty states have organ donor laws that allow you to specify the way in which you would like to help others through the use of your organs, whether by transplantation to a recipient, for scientific research, or for medical education. The magnanimous act of organ donation benefits other people either directly or indirectly.

Can my advance directive for organ donations be overridden?

The 1968 Uniform Anatomical Gift Act (on which most state donation laws are based) had no provision regarding family withdrawal of consent for an organ donation, whereas the 1987 version states that a gift not revoked by the donor before his or her death is "irrevocable and does not require the consent or concurrence of any person after the donor's death." Nevertheless, health professionals *do* ask families whether they wish to allow organ donation, and family dissent does sometimes result in a valid gift being overridden. We believe that if an individual competently consents to organ donation, and if this consent is documented on an organ donor card, it would be morally wrong for the family to attempt to overrule such a directive, and it would also be morally wrong for the health professional to honor such a request from the family. The physician can and does play a mediating role in such cases, but the physician should honor the request of the patient and should withstand coercive attempts by family members to override a valid organ donation. The physician's best response to such efforts is to educate the family about respecting the personal medical decisions made by the deceased relative and to highlight the intended altruism of the relative in donating organs after death.

What does it mean to be admitted to the intensive care unit?

When a person is admitted to an intensive care unit (or ICU) it means that the person is so severely ill that he or she requires intensive monitoring and intervention. Such monitoring may include the use of special catheters inside the large arteries or veins to monitor pressure, and the use of devices and medications to maintain blood pressure. The level of nursing attention is much greater in the ICU than the level of attention on a medical floor, because the ratio of nurses to patients is much higher.

There are many forms of medical interventions that can only be administered in the ICU. For example, because of the many complications of the therapy, some drugs in certain hospitals can only be given to patients being monitored in the ICU.

How can I decide what my preference is for an advance directive regarding ICU admission?

When you have already decided to refuse other medical therapies, you may wish to refuse to be admitted to the ICU. On the other hand, you are free to consent to ICU care for the increased attention received by patients there, while still refusing specific therapies that are used in the ICU (for example, certain drugs or the ventilator).

What does it mean to request that *911* not be called if I am at home or in a long-term care facility?

A person receiving care at home or in a nursing home (or in another long-term care setting) can direct the health care team not to take him or her to an emergency room, and not to hospitalize him or her, in the case of a sudden, worsening illness. This directive would allow the illness to run its natural course. There would be no attempt at emergency intervention by the paramedics or by health professionals at the emergency room or the hospital.

A person can refuse admission to a hospital but still request evaluation in the emergency room. If this is your wish, you should write this directive out in your Values History. Such a directive requires that the administration of any therapy being considered not entail admission to the hospital. The person is stating that, given a worsening illness, he or she does not want to be subjected to the rigors of hospitalization, even if that is the only setting in which a specific therapy can be administered. This directive does not preclude the use of other medical therapies at home or in the hospice or the long-term facility, unless the person has refused them as well, or unless they are not appropriate to the person's care.

What other advance directive options might I add to the Values History?

There are so many medical options that could be fit into this area that it may be best to agree that your agent under a durable power of attorney for health care will make such decisions. But if you feel strongly about certain therapies not specifically identified, you can state your preference in the space provided in the Values History. You may feel strongly about certain surgical interventions, or the use of certain life-prolonging medications, for example. Or you may have preferences about nursing home placement or other considerations of this kind.

You may want to request that a no-CPR order be enforced in the operating room if you are terminally ill or in a persistently vegetative state. Most surgeons and anesthesiologists prefer *not* to have a no-CPR order in the operating room; they prefer to be free to employ all possible measures to return the patient to his or her preoperative state of health. You may or may not agree with this philosophy, and you may or may not want to include this topic as a directive in your Values History.

What is proxy negation?

Proxy negation, a concept devised by Drs. Doukas and McCullough (not a standard legal term), allows you to name a person or persons openly whom you *would not want* to make decisions for you if you were unable to communicate. Such a decision is a weighty one. Your decision to name someone in this manner may arise out of your concern over conflict of interest or out of your perception that someone will attempt to request overtreatment or undertreatment of your medical condition as a result of personal conflicts, lack of communication, or differing philosophical or religious beliefs. We have found proxy negation to be appealing both to health care providers and to patients, because it attempts to exclude the voice of a designated person from consideration in a patient's care decisions, based on the patient's perception that this person will not act in accord with the patient's preferences, values, or best interest.

How will pain be treated if I'm terminally ill?

When a patient who has been diagnosed as having a terminal illness refuses life-prolonging treatment, pain control continues to be a medical concern. Even if a patient has refused other therapeutic interventions and medications, the patient is not considered to have refused pain medications. Since the intention of the doctor is to help the patient, allowing the patient to suffer pain is contrary to the doctor's goal of relieving suffering. Therefore, the doctor attempts to provide the best possible pain relief whenever pain is present during illness.

The side effects of pain medications can cause difficulties, however. Pain medicine can cause the level of breathing drive in the brain to decrease, for example. Some people are concerned that the use of pain medications during terminal illness may cause the death of the patient by interrupting this breathing drive. We believe that one must look at the intent of the pain medication, and that is to alleviate pain, not to cause the death of the patient. If we imagine ourselves suffering from a terminal form of a painful illness, such as cancer, we can see that it would be a very rational decision to want that pain controlled by whatever means necessary, even if that level of pain control might result in death. The important distinction between giving a pain medicine that may have a lethal side effect and actively killing the patient is that the intent of the former is to benefit the patient by relieving pain, while the intent of the latter is primarily to end life.

All of these medical interventions in the Values History sound painful and intrusive. Why would I even want to consider them?

Any medical therapy has the potential of benefiting you as well as the potential of harming you. What you need to weigh are, first, the level of burden you are willing to accept in receiving a therapy and, second, how much benefit you would expect from that therapy if you were unable to speak for yourself. In all cases, we believe your doctor should work with you to help you understand these therapies as well as other health care options, such as hospice care, and assure you that any pain you experience in the future will be treated with medication to alleviate your suffering.

How can I choose a therapy when I don't know what I'll be sick from?

Because people can't predict all the circumstances in which they may find themselves, many people think the best approach is to designate an agent or a proxy, someone who can make a decision based upon the circumstances existing at the time a decision must be made. But this is not always the best way to handle future uncertainty.

Although it is, of course, impossible to look into the future, many of us recognize the types of illnesses we may be susceptible to, given our family tree, our past medical history, and our past and present habits. Given this insight, it is wise, in our view, for you to provide guidance for your proxy, your family, and your doctor by stating your preferences for or against the use of the medical interventions described in the Values History. Any of the interventions described in the Values History may be required for your care someday should you become terminally ill or persistently vegetative.

In each case there are consequences to your choices. Refusal of a particular therapy may mean that the underlying disease will end your life sooner, while requesting a therapy may entail prolonging the course of that disease and extending the duration of discomfort. Further, therapies can have uncomfortable consequences, such as the trauma to your system if your body is subjected to a cardiopulmonary resuscitation. These considerations must be balanced by the consideration of whether you feel your body could survive such a therapeutic attempt if you had a terminal disease or were persistently vegetative. Only you know what is tolerable to you in terms of pain, burden, benefit, and hope. It is best to discuss considerations such as these with your doctor, who can further inform you of the medical consequences of your decisions. Sharing your medical values with your doctor will help facilitate the decision-making process.

7

You, Your Family, and Health Care Decisions

Why do *I* get to make the final decision about my advance directives?

The right to make choices about your own health care is protected *by law.* No one else can make that decision for you. Not your family, not your doctor. *No one.* If you can make a decision, or if you have already signed an advance directive or stated your concerns while competent, you can feel confident that your wishes will be followed.

Decisions about health care are deeply personal, for they have many implications for your future. Making such decisions requires self-reflection on the values you hold dear.

What if my family doesn't approve of or accept my advance directives?

Your advance directive is a legal document made *by you, for you.* No one can overrule it if you are competent when you sign it (although some states may limit the choices of advance directives available to you). Even if your family doesn't approve of an advance directive that you've signed, your word (through the directive) stands up against anyone's attempt to overrule it, including attempts by family members.

If the decisions are mine, why should I discuss them with my family?

Conflicts sometimes occur between family members about what a patient would want. That is why it is important to indicate not only what your treatment preferences are, but also who should speak for you if you are unable to speak for yourself. Once you have decided who that person will be, you should discuss your preferences and values very carefully with him or her. You also should explain, briefly, to your family why you have chosen the person or persons named as your proxies, and describe in general what decisions you have asked them to make. It is a good idea to write some of this information down. The written explanation will help your agent deal with family members or others who may not fully understand your wishes.

Explaining your preferences in advance helps people to accept them when the time comes. It also avoids misinterpretation of your preferences. For example, an ethical quandary often arises after a relative arrives on the hospital scene to see the now ill and noncommunicative patient. The relative, who may not have communicated with the patient for a long time, then orders that "everything possible be done." Regardless of his or her love and devotion for the patient (and perhaps guilt over family issues that the medical team doesn't know about), this relative is making the waters murky, not clarifying them.

Avoid such scenarios by clearly communicating your preferences to your doctor and family. Be sure to discuss which therapies you would consider futile in specific circumstances.

Is this why it's important for me to name a proxy?

Yes. The family member, friend, or loved one with whom you have discussed your values, beliefs, and preferences will be able to make decisions based on *what you would want.* They will be choosing medical therapies when you are unable to speak for yourself. You'll want them to choose what you would have chosen had you been able to communicate your wishes.

When considering using a proxy, the essential component is *communication.* Communication between patient and family or other agent must be reliable and preferably will be ongoing, so that your proxy's understanding reflects your current thinking. It's best to have frank and open conversations with the rest of the family now, so that there are no misconceptions concerning what you would want in the way of medical care. This prevents the values and beliefs of the rest of your family from interfering with your wishes, which are based on your own values and beliefs. There is little benefit in naming a proxy to act on your behalf and then not discussing your medical values and health care preferences with that individual.

Why does interpersonal conflict occur?

Interpersonal conflict occurs when there is a difference of opinion or values between two persons, both of whom may believe they are acting in the patient's interest. This can happen within the family when the patient has a specific set of values and beliefs that conflicts with the values and beliefs of someone else within the family. It usually occurs when there is a difference of opinion regarding what constitutes overtreatment or undertreatment.

Sometimes a family member wishes to initiate treatment or continue to treat because the relative so deeply wants the patient to continue living that he or she either doesn't look closely at the preferences of the patient or believes that these stated preferences don't represent what the patient would really want. Also, it is possible that a conflict of interest—due to ill will, for example, or concern about cost or burden of care, or a desire to receive an inheritance—may prompt a family member to undertreat an incapacitated person. In any of these instances, a family member might wish for the patient to be undertreated, regardless of the patient's desire for continued treatment.

As family physicians, we have encountered many family conflicts. These emotional interpersonal conflicts may be brought to a head when the family is burdened with the stress of a dying or persistently vegetative patient. Advance directives are very helpful in preventing or minimizing such conflicts, because decisions regarding your health care will already have been made—*by you.* Otherwise, your doctor will have to sort through the many emotions and agendas within your family to determine who might best speak for you. In our experience, this latter way of making these important decisions does a disservice to your family, your doctor, and, most importantly, you.

Whom can I appoint to speak for me?

You can transfer the right of making decisions to someone in your family or to a friend or loved one, as we have discussed before, with the durable power of attorney for health care. Several states have living will laws that allow for the naming of a proxy (you'll need to consult your own state's laws to determine whether your state permits this). You can also hold informal conversations with others. These conversations can prove valuable in their discussions with the health care team, should decisions about your health care need to be made.

Your agent must not have any conflict of interest regarding the decisions he or she must make. He or she is responsible for conveying your values and preferences when you are no longer able to speak, and his or her values, beliefs, financial concerns, or other interests must not present a conflict of interest that could affect your care adversely.

Can I appoint my doctor to speak for me?

No. Having your doctor serve as your proxy or agent would be inappropriate, since the doctor is the one trying to do his or her best to manage your health care. There is also a possibility of a conflict of interest between what the doctor would want to do and what you would want done for yourself, or what your family members would want done for you. The potential conflict lies in the balance between the responsibility of the doctor to heal and minimize harm and the responsibility to respect your advance directives or proxy consent. The direct conflict of interest between these two principles makes it impossible for one person to fulfill both roles.

Can a family speak for a patient if the patient did not execute an advance directive?

In some states the family can do so even when no advance directive has been signed by the patient. Several states have statutes that allow a family member to speak for the patient even without a durable power of attorney for health care. Even in those states, however, if you want a *specific* person to make your health care decisions, you must name your agent or proxy explicitly through a durable power of attorney for health care.

In states without such laws, the family will be included in discussions about the patient's treatment but the doctors are not legally obligated to follow the family's instructions. Nevertheless, families should aim to guide the patient's health care based as much as possible on the general values and beliefs of the patient rather than on their own preferences. In this way, the family can actively advocate the patient's belief system when the patient is unable to talk for himself or herself. Ultimately, this concept was of critical importance to the Nancy Cruzan case (discussed in chapter 8).

Sometimes family members don't agree about what a patient would want under the circumstances presented. To prevent conflicts, as we have stressed throughout this book, it is best to document your medical preferences now. People who have conversations with their families about their values and preferences (after signing an advance directive) can feel confident that their wishes will be carried out in the future. Through these conversations, family members gain an insight into each other, and this knowledge will make it easier for them to speak for each other if the need ever presents itself.

What issues should I discuss with my proxy or agent?

In addition to medical preferences, you may want to discuss your general values, your religious values, and your philosophical values. Having an understanding of your values will be very helpful to your family if you are unable to speak for yourself. These values are of particular importance when medical events don't occur as you had anticipated. Holding open-ended discussions about your values allows your family to better understand what you would want done if they ever need to make decisions for you.

A discussion of your values may include issues such as where you would like to live and how you would like to be cared for should you become frail or incapacitated. Choices concerning home health care, assisted living, and nursing home placement can be discussed. You may want to state your preferences among the alternatives that are available for nursing home care, specifying, for example, what kind of environment you would prefer. You may also address what form of religious or memorial service (if any) you would want performed after your death, and you may state your preferences regarding burial, cremation, or donation of your body.

What happens if I become unable to speak for myself and I haven't yet discussed my medical values and preferences?

Someone will have to make these decisions for you. If you have not discussed your values or preferences, and if you have not executed a written directive, members of your family (or someone else) may have to make decisions based on what they *think* would be in your best interest. Their judgment may not be the same as yours. By not signing an advance directive, you may burden not only your family (who will have to make painful decisions for you without the benefit of insight into your preferences) but yourself, for you may be subjected to treatments that you don't want. Again, it is best to have discussions with your family, friends, and physicians as soon as possible.

What if I have these discussions but there are conflicting opinions about my care within my family when I cannot speak for myself?

Conflicts within families can become a real problem when there are preexisting difficulties in family dynamics. Different family members may give conflicting opinions about your care, all of them believing that what they say reflects your wishes and is in your best interest. These opinions may be based on a misunderstanding of your past statements concerning your wishes or values about health care; they may be held out of a loving concern to keep you alive at all costs (regardless of your past wishes); or they may arise without any regard for your best interests—they may be the result of a direct conflict of interest. As noted above, interpersonal conflicts can occur between family members because of any number of emotional, behavioral, and monetary motives. Such conflicts can wreak havoc on the family's attempts to make decisions on behalf of a person who can no longer speak for himself or herself. That is why it is best to name (and document through a durable power of attorney for health care) the person whom you want to make the decisions. It is also why written preferences are critical in helping your proxy make the decisions he or she must make.

What if my doctor suspects a conflict of interest on the part of my agent or proxy?

If the physician suspects a conflict of interest on the part of your proxy concerning what would be best for you, the physician can call on other members of the family in consultation to try to reach a consensus within the family, or, in most hospitals and some nursing homes, the physician can call on an ethics committee for advice to help decide how best to treat you. Consultations by ethics committees allow for deliberations on medical cases that present a moral conflict. If this option is not available, the courts may become an arbiter in cases where conflicting medical viewpoints are heard; the legal ruling that results in these cases *must* be carried out.

What is a guardian or conservator?

A guardian or conservator is a person appointed by the court to take care of another person who has been deemed unable to make decisions for himself or herself.

A guardian may be given authority to make all kinds of decisions (financial, personal, and business), or the guardian's authority may be limited by the court to a specific area (the financial, for example). Depending on your state's laws, you may be allowed to specify whom you might want (or not want) to serve as your guardian in the future.

Do advance directives make it unnecessary for a guardian to be assigned?

Because advance directives, particularly durable powers of attorney, allow you to state your own decisions regarding health care, you won't need to have a guardian appointed to make health care decisions for you in the future. A durable power of attorney for health care also will be helpful to a judge who must decide whom to appoint if you need a guardian for other purposes. The durable power of attorney for health care, the living will, and the Values History—all can enhance medical decision making in case of your future incapacity, so that the need for a guardian for medical decisions might be eliminated.

8

Signing Advance Directives

Why should I consider signing an advance directive now?

It's a fallacy to believe you can wait until you're approaching the end of your life to make advance directive decisions. Illness or accidents can happen *to anyone at any time*. Nancy Cruzan, for example, was only in her twenties when she had an accident that left her in a persistently vegetative state. (Her family's difficult situation is described in the pages that follow.) For this reason, we believe that adults need to make these advance directive decisions as soon as they can bring themselves to think about them. Otherwise, the family or the courts may be forced to make these decisions on their behalf in the future.

Why has the subject of advance directives recently received so much attention?

The attention of the nation was focused on this issue in 1991 by a landmark case decided by the Supreme Court. This case involved a young woman, Nancy Cruzan, who had been injured in an auto accident at the age of 26 that left her in a persistently vegetative state. The Cruzan family asked the U.S. Supreme Court to consider the case after the state supreme court in their home state of Missouri ruled against the family's wishes to withdraw the gastrostomy tube that had been providing life-sustaining nutrition and hydration for Nancy for six years. The Missouri Supreme Court ruled that Nancy Cruzan's oral wishes concerning medical care, which she had discussed with family and friends, did not constitute "clear and convincing evidence" of her intent. The U.S. Supreme Court upheld the right of the state of Missouri to require "clear and convincing" evidence but did not require that the evidence be in writing.

The U.S. Supreme Court's ruling in the *Cruzan* case gave great weight to the right of individuals to refuse life-sustaining medical therapy, including nutrition and hydration. Further, Justice Sandra Day O'Connor's opinion brought attention to the fact that people do not take adequate advantage of opportunities to express themselves through a living will or durable power of attorney. For example, had Nancy Cruzan executed a durable power of attorney for health care, the family likely would have been able to carry out her stated wishes and discontinue use of the gastrostomy tube.

Several months after the Supreme Court ruling, new witnesses, previously unknown to the Cruzan family, came forward to offer corroborating testimony that Nancy Cruzan would not want to live on a feeding tube in a persistently vegetative state. With this testimony, which the trial court found to be "clear and convincing," Nancy Cruzan finally had her preference—to discontinue therapy—honored.

Is age a factor in considering advance directives?

It seems natural that the younger and healthier the individual, the more likely that individual is to postpone preparing an advance directive. Yet, many young adults have accidents that leave them permanently disabled. We ask the participants in our educational programs whether they have an advance directive, and usually a majority of them, whether they are young or old, health professionals or not, indicate that they have *not* prepared any type of directive.

Because of the Patient Self-Determination Act, young adults and older adults will be given information about an advance directive upon admittance to a hospital, nursing home, hospice, home health agency, or health maintenance organization. Therefore, we can anticipate that more members of all age groups will begin thinking about these options.

In the *Cruzan* case, the family and friends of Nancy Cruzan provided testimony that she had expressed her values on medical care when she was well. The Missouri Supreme Court did not recognize this testimony because the trial court had not described it as "clear and convincing." The U.S. Supreme Court ruled that Missouri could require "clear and convincing evidence" that Nancy Cruzan would want her feeding tubes withdrawn. We anticipate that, together, the decision in *Cruzan* and the Patient Self-Determination Act will inspire many people, young *and* old, to attend to the preparation of an advance directive. That is our hope. There is no doubt in our minds that an advance directive provides clear and convincing evidence of a person's wishes.

In advance directive counseling and care, what differences can we expect according to age?

It seems likely that the middle-aged and elderly will be thinking more about the possible need for an advance directive and will have more frequent contacts with the medical care system, through office visits to the doctor, hospitalizations, and nursing home admissions. The elderly may hear more about living wills and durable powers of attorney for health care in efforts directed to the "senior citizen" population, from presentations by state and local offices on aging, or within retirement communities. *All* adults are candidates for advance directives, however.

The elderly will not be the only age group approached about advance directives, though, for the young will confront the advance directive issue, too. On admittance to a health maintenance organization or whenever they are hospitalized for any reason, they will hear about this option for advance planning. Just as the elderly will be informed in many ways, and just as physicians will be kept up to date through educational sessions and review of procedural guidelines, the young will hear about advance directives, too.

We anticipate a process of cultural change in which young adults, for example, on an initial visit to a health maintenance organization for the purpose of giving a medical history and having a physical examination, will receive literature on the subject and be asked to think about their values, beliefs, and choices so these ideas can be developed into an advance directive during a future set of visits. Although advance directives will more likely affect the lives of the chronically and acutely ill (and therefore mostly elderly people), we anticipate that advance directives will soon be understood as being beneficial for the entire society.

Are there different considerations for the young and old?

Many older persons seem to be more accepting of death than younger persons. They may demonstrate attitudes that are more accepting, reflecting a sense of anticipatory readiness. Many chronically ill people wonder why they are still here, or why they are still alive. People who are ill and are confined to hospitals or long-term care facilities, and people who are less active and have already given up much of their former independence, may demonstrate the greatest acceptance or readiness. Many older people are comforted by religious beliefs that help them look forward to their impending death.

In general, the elderly who are closest to death are more comfortable with the notion of death than those who are furthest from it; those who are furthest from death are less accepting and show greater denial and anger. The young man or woman who suddenly becomes terminally ill with a malignancy or AIDS will generally (and, it would seem, naturally) be in a much greater state of shock than the person in his or her eighties who has been chronically ill with congestive heart failure and emphysema, and who has had repeated hospitalizations over the past several years. The sixteenth-century French essayist Michel de Montaigne wrote that we could not endure sudden deterioration. "But," he wrote, "when we are led by Nature's hand down a gentle and virtually imperceptible slope, bit by bit, one step at a time, she rolls us into this wretched state and makes us familiar with it."

Do the issues that enter a person's Values History or advance directive change as a person ages?

It is certainly possible that one's choices in the living will or durable power of attorney or Values History may change over time. As noted above, the younger person who is seriously ill may be in a state of shock, while the chronically ill elderly person who has been combating various health problems and declining over a period of years may be more accepting of death. They will both bring emotionally laden concerns to the process of wanting to complete an advance directive.

The ideal time for every adult to prepare the advance directive, whether living will, durable power of attorney for health care, or the Values History, is *when the individual is well.* It is best to sign advance directives after having taken time to reflect on the directives and having had discussions with family members and friends, your minister or spiritual advisor, your lawyer, and, particularly, your doctor. It's true that such a directive should be reevaluated periodically, in the same fashion that the will for one's financial estate should be reevaluated.

Why can't all this wait until later?

You never know when you suddenly will be unable to speak for yourself. Also, advance directives allow for decisions to be made on your behalf if you become incapacitated *temporarily* (for example, after an accident or surgery). By confronting the task of reflecting on your values and signing an advance directive now, you safeguard your right to control your health care in a way that no other present mechanism can. In this way, your ability to have therapies begun or discontinued will be facilitated if you are ever unable to speak for yourself. The vast majority of deaths occur in the hospital or the nursing home; but this is not the place or time to reflect on your values and execute an advance directive. It is in your best interest to sign an advance directive *now*, rather than wait until you're admitted into a health care institution.

We must all appreciate that it is often hard to make such decisions when illness is not present and we are still fully competent. It is difficult to imagine the prospect of losing the ability to make our own medical decisions. We all demonstrate some denial, procrastination, and indecision. Understanding these human characteristics should make us feel less guilty, but we must nevertheless realize the importance of getting started and acting now.

Can't I just count on my family to decide?

That's a fairly heavy burden to place on someone else. This responsibility is best exercised by you directly, for your sake and for the sake of your family. Once you have made your own decisions, your family is freed from ever having to guess what decision you would make. Also, as we saw in the *Cruzan* case, the courts may require clear and convincing evidence of your preferences, at least regarding termination of care.

What about active euthanasia and assisted suicide?

The subjects of euthanasia (or mercy killing) and assisted suicide have become more visible in the public and professional literature and have captured the attention of the public. These subjects have been brought to the public's attention by the Kevorkian "death machine"; the assisted suicide "Quill" case in Rochester, New York; the (failed) Washington State initiative; Derek Humphrey's book *Final Exit;* and publicity surrounding the Dutch practice of permitting euthanasia (when the patient *competently* requests it).

Why do you think there is increased interest in euthanasia and assisted suicide?

Almost everyone is concerned about the use of sophisticated technology on persons with advanced illness. Although modern treatments are often helpful, there is increasing concern from patients about the effort and the cost in physical, financial, and emotional terms during the last months of life when there is little benefit in such treatment. Many elderly people are angered by what they perceive as life-sustaining measures that are invasive, burdensome, and futile, and therefore they are searching for other alternatives.

What's the difference between active euthanasia and passive euthanasia?

In much of the public discussion, there is confusion related to the failure to distinguish between active euthanasia (or so-called mercy killing, in which measures are taken that directly and actively cause the patient's death) and passive euthanasia (which refers to the withdrawal of treatments provided to the terminally ill or persistently vegetative patient). The public is done a great disservice when the terms *active euthanasia* and *passive euthanasia* are used interchangeably, either by the media or in doctor-patient discussions.

Active euthanasia can either be voluntary (in which the patient freely consents to actions that will cause his or her death) or involuntary (in which someone else, such as a family member or doctor, makes this decision). In either circumstance, active euthanasia represents a profound change in the doctor-patient relationship. The physician who participates in a mercy killing faces moral and legal issues very different from those faced by the physician who allows a patient to refuse treatments knowing that the refusal will result in death. In active euthanasia or mercy killing, the intent is to cause death, with immediate cessation of life resulting from a single act. In passive euthanasia, when the patient allows life-supporting measures to be withdrawn, the disease itself causes death.

Another distinction (discussed in chapter 6) is made between administering a drug to cause death and using a medication with the intention of alleviating pain and suffering, even if the medication may have the additional effect of shortening life. Most people agree that the latter is far different from mercy killing or assisted suicide.

What can we learn from the practice of euthanasia in the Netherlands?

Recent accounts from the Netherlands, where active euthanasia requested by the patient is tolerated, indicate that many of the patients who died as a result of active euthanasia had not explicitly requested this action. It is our opinion that the patient's autonomy may not be adequately safeguarded in the present Dutch system.

Both the decision in *Cruzan* and the Patient Self-Determination Act have provided the impetus for an ideal system, one in which adult Americans state their autonomous wishes, their values, and their self-determination. In this system, respect for patient rights to consent and refuse care rightly dominate the discussion, and issues swirling around the concerns of active euthanasia are not a focus.

What alternatives exist to the practices of euthanasia and assisted suicide?

What all people want as we confront life and death, and what we as physicians believe would arrest the demands for mercy killing and assisted suicide, are, first, alleviation of pain and suffering; second, avoidance of futile and burdensome technologies that do not benefit the patient; and, third, a physician who will provide strength, support, and comfort. As physicians and as members of a larger community, we can provide the rational alternative to mercy killing and assisted suicide, by allowing patients the option of "dying well" (a phrase used in the literature by Dr. Arthur J. Dyck and Dr. William Reichel).

Physicians, nurses, and other health professionals involved in primary care medicine already provide comprehensive care, paying attention to the family and the home, and taking psychosocial issues into account. Your own primary care physician—whether a family physician or an internist—can better help you to "die well." Helping a patient "die well" not only is a function of the physician's abilities to relieve pain and suffering, but also relates to having respect for a dying patient's choices and wishes and values as expressed when ill and dying, or as stated in an advance directive or by means of the patient's proxy.

The widespread use of advance directives may very well bring about revolutionary change. For example, many individuals now choose to die at home rather than in a hospital or nursing home as the illness reaches a point of finality. Supporting this decision is the success of the hospice movement, which emphasizes home care, as well as significant technological and pharmacological advances, including improved knowledge and techniques for pain management in the home care setting. We can envision the hopelessly ill patient, young or old, choosing to remain at home in the advanced stages of illness, receiving care from family and friends, and having steadfast support and comfort provided by a physician, a nurse, and others.

Are there religious or spiritual considerations in the use of advance directives?

Considering the diversities of religious belief and experience in the United States, one can well imagine that some people may have a problem with advance directives, including living wills and durable powers of attorney for health care. Some may believe that any attempt to withhold a life-supporting therapy, particularly nutrition, is wrong. Others may worry that living wills and other advance directives create a "slippery slope" that leads to active euthanasia and assisted suicide. However, most people believe strongly, as we do, that living wills, durable powers of attorney for health care, and, in particular, the Values History, promote individual freedom to stop therapies that are futile for the treatment of illness rather than encourage active euthanasia and suicide. Rejecting practices that intentionally cause the cessation of life (such as active euthanasia and assisted suicide), the informed individual can at the same time reject burdensome, invasive, and futile treatments by making certain decisions in advance. Discussing these decisions with your religious adviser may ease your mind; such a discussion allows you to reflect openly on the spiritual reasons for your choices.

We have met many elderly people who have strong religious beliefs affirming God or acknowledging the presence of a higher power or the Lord in their lives, and who suffer with health problems with dignity and serenity. These individuals have no problem in stating their wishes and requests with great equanimity. They have lived a full life and, having accepted the possibility of death, have written an advance directive.

The patient who affirms the presence of God in his or her life is empowered to make choices for palliative or comfort care and to make his or her wishes or choices known in advance. These choices may include rejecting life-sustaining therapies if the burdens of illness and the burdens of therapies cross a certain threshold.

Of course, there is a fine line between treatments that will benefit the patient and the treatments that are burdensome and futile. Ideally, there is an ongoing, intimate dialogue between the individual and the doctor, so that each stage of the illness and treatment is evaluated and reevaluated. The patient may have survived many crises in which he or she benefited from medical therapy. With the illness advancing, the patient may feel that another round of invasive treatment for coronary artery disease, or another attempt at chemotherapy or radiation therapy for advanced malignancy, is simply beyond what he or she wants. At that point, the patient or his or her proxy designate may ask for comfort or palliative care. Some or all medications may be discontinued, and an intravenous drip might be continued with morphine to reduce pain, such as in the case of advanced cancer, or to relieve severe congestive heart failure. The purpose of the morphine is not to end life but to keep the person comfortable.

In considering terminal illness, what is the role of hospice care?

Hospice care developed first in England (particularly at St. Christopher's Hospice under Dr. Cicely Saunders) and then moved to the United States, first to New Haven, Connecticut, in the mid 1970s, and then gradually throughout the country. The person accepted for hospice is usually not expected to survive beyond a six-month period. The patient's physician is called upon to certify that the person likely will die within six months according to the natural course of the illness.

Hospice care is a philosophy of management of pain and suffering associated with dying. The palliative or comfort care manages the patient's pain, using pain medications in amounts necessary to guarantee that the patient is pain free. Clinical strategies or treatments that could prolong life are stopped.

The hospice focuses on the family or others who are providing care, as well as on the dying person. This includes paying attention to the psychological, social, and spiritual aspects of care. In some circumstances hospice services are available around the clock, seven days per week.

Hospice care may be carried out at home, in hospice beds in hospitals and nursing homes, or in free-standing hospices. There are many variations of hospice care in the United States. Some hospices are part of home health agencies or work in parallel with a home health agency, providing special focus on hospice principles. The hospice provides case management and follows the patient as he or she might move back and forth between home and inpatient facilities. If necessary to improve control of pain and other symptoms, the hospice may place the dying person in an inpatient setting. If the dying person's needs simply cannot be handled by the caregivers at home, the hospice will place the dying person in a hospice bed.

Who are the members of the hospice team?

Although hospice allows continuity of care between the home and other inpatient settings, the patient's personal physician often does not play the key medical role. Often the hospice physician takes charge medically. Alternatively, the patient's personal physician may work with the hospice team, backing up the nursing staff with telephone consultation and speaking with the patient and the family by telephone.

Every member of the team—physician, nurse, social worker and chaplain—is familiar with hospice principles. Hospice workers are highly skilled in methods of pain control and in working with terminally ill persons and their families. Hospice physicians and nurses have knowledge and skill in these areas that may not be found in the general medical and nursing community. We can expect that in the future, medical and nursing education in medical schools, residency training programs, nursing schools, and continuing education programs will pay greater attention to hospice principles than has been paid to date.

Hospice has also created an army of trained volunteers who provide support for the patient and the family. A hospice volunteer's ability to enhance care, support, and comfort is remarkable. Many hospices also offer support groups for families facing the loss of their loved one. For more information about hospice care, or to locate a hospice in your area, write the National Hospice Organization at 1901 North Moore Street, Suite 901, Arlington, Virginia 22209, or call 703/243-5900.

Will my physician be willing to collaborate with me to develop an advance directive?

Because of the *Cruzan* decision and the Patient Self-Determination Act, physicians will rapidly become increasingly familiar with living wills, durable powers of attorney for health care, and other advance directives. Despite the findings of the national living will survey (discussed in chapter 5), things are changing, and many forces will work to involve the physician more actively in the preparation and use of advance directives.

The physician is in the best position to discuss these matters, because he or she knows more about the person's health and illness, and what scenarios are possible, than anyone. The physician also understands the importance of the many medical terms: dementia, coma, persistently vegetative state, heart attack, ischemic heart disease and congestive heart disease, stroke, malignancy, and so on. The physician understands the use and implications of life-supporting therapies: ventilators, feeding tubes, dialysis, antibiotics, and cardiopulmonary resuscitation. Again, the discussion of an advance directive such as the Values History would best take place in the physician's office over a period of time.

Presently, there may be many forces working against the physician's active participation. Traditionally, for example, physicians have not spent time on advance directives but have concentrated on the treatment of illnesses such as bronchitis or diabetes, or on preventive medicine such as cholesterol reduction or Pap smears. The physician feels time pressures. Increasingly, too, corporate and managed health care systems (such as health maintenance organizations and preferred provider organizations) are concerned with productivity. Also, physicians differ when it comes to values, attitudes, beliefs, and behaviors. For example, some are more interested in the organic, and others are more interested in a broader, "biopsychosocial model" of health. A physician may be so preoccupied with the patient's chief complaint (for example, fatigue) that handling the patient's medical problems may consume all of his or her thoughts. Thinking and talking about possible future medical scenarios and advance directives may not occur to the busy, preoccupied physician.

Another factor that works against physician participation is that no official billing method exists to reimburse physicians for counseling a patient regarding the development of an advance directive. Under Medicare and many other health insurance plans, the physician must include counseling under another reason for the visit, such as high blood pressure, to be reimbursed by a third-party payer such as Medicare or Blue Cross/Blue Shield.

Until now, the physician simply may not have been sufficiently familiar with living wills and advance directives, or may not have been sufficiently interested to serve as an advocate for this growing movement, to encourage patients to develop such a document. Other demands placed on the physician may have prevented this task from rising to the top of the doctor's priorities. Some physicians, however, have systematically sent letters to their entire practice; in the letter the physicians offer a model living will, durable power of attorney for health care, or advance directive, and invite the patient to come in to the office to discuss the matter. This is a very good sign.

Many other physicians have received the living will or

durable power of attorney for health care from the patient and have simply placed it in the patient's chart for safekeeping without discussion. The physician should commend the patient for completing the document, thoroughly discuss the patient's decision and his or her understanding of it, and then file the directive. (On receiving and filing a directive, physicians should identify the file's contents by marking the outside of the patient's folder with a label that says: PATIENT'S LIVING WILL, DURABLE POWER OF ATTORNEY, OR ADVANCE DIRECTIVE IS FILED IN THIS CHART. The label also ought to state the date when the directive was received.)

While it is true that many physicians have not yet approached this new social trend with great energy or enthusiasm, few would openly reject a directive and express a negative philosophy on the matter. By discussing living wills, durable powers of attorney, and advance directives with your physician, you will gain insight into your physician's attitudes, values, and behavior regarding the role of advance directives in his or her practice.

The future looks even brighter. Medical schools and residency training programs are now focusing on medical ethics—and particularly decision making around the end of life. Since passage of the Patient Self-Determination Act, too, physicians in practice are being offered workshops by the hospital medical staffs to which they belong and other sources, such as managed health care programs. Advance directives are turning up as a prominent topic in the major medical journals and at continuing medical education courses. It is to be hoped that a long-term effect of the Act will be a wider acceptance of advance directives by physicians and their patients.

What if the physician objects to the decision called for by the advance directive or the proxy?

A major difficulty that physicians may have with advance directives or proxies and living wills is the potential for conflict between the dictates of an advance directive or proxy decision maker and the physician's opinion in a given case. For example, suppose the physician senses intuitively that this patient can be helped with surgery or other therapies. The physician may say that he or she wants to be governed by the patient's circumstances, not by a piece of paper. Some may say that patients cannot fully anticipate what their preference would be in a specific medical scenario, or that patients simply know too little about these matters to make decisions in advance. But these objections only add credence to the argument for physician training. The physician needs to learn how to educate the patient and how, through competent counseling, he or she can learn what the patient's values, attitudes, and choices are, as well as how to respect them. It is essential that competent people know that their wishes, not the wishes of a caring, paternalistic physician, will be implemented in the future.

Suppose the physician recently lost a patient who could have been saved had the physician not followed the patient's advance directives. Might that experience affect how closely the physician follows the next patient's advance directives? It shouldn't. Suppose a patient has become mentally incompetent since preparing an advance directive one year earlier, when he or she was fully competent. Might the physician say that, under the new circumstances, the previously stated wishes, choices, and directives are no longer valid? The physician shouldn't.

Suppose the physician receives overwhelming pressure from the family to reverse the preferences of the patient, as stated in a competently written advance directive. Should the physician succumb to this pressure and overrule the patient's wishes? The physician shouldn't. Physicians are not to impose their desire to benefit the hopelessly ill patient with a specific treatment (under the guise of beneficence) and disregard advance directives that were clearly stated just because the physician (or the family) believes that under the current circumstances the patient might want to change his or her choice or preference.

The future should certainly build the necessary advance directive counseling skills into the medical education and the continuing education of the physician. The future should certainly provide for reimbursement to the physician who provides this counseling. Future standards of care should require review of these issues on a timely basis, just as the regularly performed Pap smear and cholesterol measurement are standards of good care.

What if my doctor doesn't condone advance directives?

Your physician has an ethical and, in most states, a legal obligation either to follow your advance directive or to transfer your medical care to another doctor who will be able to follow the decisions, including refusal of care, that you've documented in your advance directive.

What if I change my mind about part of my advance directive?

As we have mentioned before, because this is a possibility, the advance directive should be reviewed periodically in the same fashion that a will providing for the disposition of a financial estate should be reviewed. Our experience suggests that people's choices are fairly stable from year to year. Nevertheless, we recommend that the physician make a point of re-examining advance directives with the patient on a regular basis. *You are free to change or revoke your previous treatment directives at any time.*

What is the best advance directive method?

Each has its own merits, and we do not favor one specific method over another. Living wills are designed primarily to provide for refusal of life-sustaining treatment should you become terminally ill, but several states allow its use for a person in a persistently vegetative state. The living will allows you to articulate directly (rather than through another person) your autonomous preferences, following specific instructions appended to the document (as allowed by most states).

A durable power of attorney for health care applies to any kind of medical decision that might need to be made if you are unable to communicate, whether or not you are terminally ill. It permits you to designate a decision maker and to specify the kinds of treatments you *do* want as well as those you *do not* want. Your agent or proxy can follow your instructions in the future.

The Values History is a powerful adjunct to both of

these documents. It allows you to identify your medical values as well as the specific medical treatments you would accept or refuse.

Step by step, how should I document my wishes using the advance directives you've mentioned?

You can state your wishes about terminal illness through a living will and provide details about your medical values and advance directives through the Values History. These documents can be supplemented by the durable power of attorney for health care, which appoints an agent whose role is to make certain that your preferences are implemented by your doctor. This approach focuses on treatment refusal in case of terminal illness. An alternative approach is to sign a durable power of attorney for health care and to supplement it with a Values History and a living will (for emphasis and to guide your agent).

When you work with your attorney to draw up a will or trust for estate purposes, your attorney may bring up the subject of advance directives. If he or she does not, you should ask your attorney about the various options of advance directives available in your state. If the attorney who usually handles your affairs is not up to date on advance directives, our advice is to seek the advice of a local attorney who is very familiar with the laws in your state.

If you want to fill out your advance directives without an attorney, you have several options. First, you can obtain a living will or durable power of attorney (usually for free) from a variety of sources: your own family doctor, your local hospital administration office, your state attorney general's office, your health maintenance organization, your local state representative, the citizen advocate group called Choice in Dying, or the American Association of Retired Persons. After receiving a copy of the living will and durable power of attorney for health care, you should make photocopies of the blank forms for all adult members of your family.

Second, we recommend that you sit down with your doctor to discuss the meaning of signing these documents. You may want to make sure that plenty of time is scheduled for this component of your next medical visit when you make your appointment. Your doctor will be able to answer any questions you might have about the use or refusal of life-sustaining medical therapies. You should ask your doctor whether and when he or she would honor your right to refuse certain treatments.

You should make sure that the person you wish to speak for you agrees to serve as your agent in a durable power of attorney for health care. This is a role with the potential for significant responsibility, and the person ought to understand the significance of the role before agreeing to serve. It is also prudent to select an alternative proxy who would serve if your first choice were unable to fulfill the task. Finally, after you have had these discussions and you have decided what your preferences are, you can fill out the forms. Sign the forms in the presence of two witnesses. *Be careful not to sign the advance directive until your two witnesses are present.*

At this point you should make copies: one for your doctor's medical records, one for your agent, and one for each family member with whom you want to share this information. Extra copies should be made for good measure. If you are ever hospitalized, and the hospital (in keeping with the Patient Self-Determination Act) asks you if you have an advance directive, you can now answer yes, and you can ask a family member to bring a copy to be included in the hospital's medical record.

As a next step in the advance directive process, we recommend that you make a copy of the Values History found in the Appendix of this book. At this point, you may want to talk with your doctor, your spouse, and other family members about the values you consider important. These discussions need not be rushed—you can discuss your values and preferences with your family, friends, or religious adviser over several months, and you can talk with your doctor over the course of several visits. This process will be most productive for you if it is reflective and introspective. You will know the best way—your own way—to complete this process.

When you are ready, fill out the Values Section of the Values History, detailing those values that would be most important in your care if you were terminally ill or persistently vegetative. Also, explain why or in what way these values are important to you and your medical decision making. If you are presently ill, you may already have strong feelings in this regard. Write them down. This written record will let other people know about your medical values and how you wish them to influence your care in the future.

After you have completed the Values Section, continue on to the Directives Section of the Values History. Before completing this section, review the medical interventions most relevant to your medical condition with your family doctor. For instance, a person with known chronic lung disease may have very strong feelings about being placed on a ventilator, particularly if this person has been placed on a ventilator in the past. By reviewing all of these directives you have a much better chance of accomplishing what a living will is intended to accomplish: completing an informed consent to request or refuse life-sustaining treatments.

In this section, you can specify which health care options you definitely would—or would not—select for yourself, by marking them in the appropriate places. If you would like to specify a trial of intervention for specific health care options (as discussed in chapter 6), indicate that this is your preference; you can choose either a time-limited trial or a trial based on medically judged benefit. Remember that the option of a trial of intervention based on medically judged benefit requires a great deal of communication between you, your doctor, and your proxy to establish a clear understanding of your values and preferences. The space for "other" directives at the end of the Directives Section allows you to specify other medical therapeutic options whose use you wish to consent to or to refuse.

If there are family members or other persons whom you want to disqualify from making decisions for you, those persons should be identified in the proxy negation section of the Values History. This directive informs your family, your agent for durable power of attorney for health care, and your family doctor about the absence of standing this individual has regarding your care.

You may also at this time wish to fill out an organ donor card, available from the department of motor vehicles in most states, so that if you die and your organs are still useful, you may give a gift of life to another. Giving such a gift is a truly heroic and altruistic act.

Once you have completed the Values History (again, this may take some time and several office visits), we recommend that you photocopy the completed Values History and give a copy to your agent or agents, those individuals named in your durable power of attorney for health care. Along with your Values History, again, be sure to give your agent a copy of your living will and your instructions (if any) in your durable power of attorney for health care. These documents will make it easier for someone to make decisions on your behalf if you ever are unable to speak for yourself, because your values and your treatment preferences are clearly described. Any unforeseen medical circumstances will be much more easily resolved.

Also give a copy of the completed Values History to your doctor.

Keep the original copy of your living will, durable power of attorney for health care, and Values History in a safe and accessible place in your home, so they will be quickly available should you become ill. *Do not put your advance directives in your safe deposit box,* because no one will be able to get them if you become incapacitated.

You now have a very powerful set of documents to speak on your behalf should you ever be unable to make your own health care decisions or speak for yourself.

Why should I consider signing a living will when I could just sign a durable power of attorney for health care?

The durable power of attorney for health care is an important advance directive, but not everyone has a relative or friend whom they would feel comfortable appointing as a proxy decision maker. And not everyone has a surviving relative or close friend to consider for this role.

The living will allows you to express your preferences and eliminates the need for a proxy decision maker. With a living will, even if you cannot chose a proxy, you are still able to choose your own preferences for your future health care.

What should I do if there is no official living will or durable power of attorney for health care law in my state?

Because each state has its own laws regarding the use of advance directives, living wills, and durable powers of attorney, we recommend that you prepare these documents with the assistance of a local attorney who is well versed in the laws in your state regarding these advance directives. The generic living will and durable power of attorney for health care which are reproduced in the Appendix might serve as a starting point for your own thoughts, your discussions with your family, and your formal discussions with your physician and attorney. It is important to note that these generic forms may not be legally binding in your state.

How should I think through my decisions?

It's probably best to think through the issues involved in advance directives over a period of time. It probably is not prudent to consider these important issues quickly, just to get something down on paper. We recommend that you reflect on these decisions for several weeks or months before putting them down on paper.

Will I feel "settled" when I sign an advance directive?

In our experience, people who sign a living will or a durable power of attorney feel much more settled about the kinds of things that might happen should they be unable to speak for themselves. Having these preferences written down, and feeling confident that they will be respected, puts your mind at ease. Knowing that these decisions will not be left to other people, such as your doctor or your family, and that your wishes will be followed even if you are unable to talk, can be a great comfort.

Advance directives are an important part of future planning. They are best completed now, in the present, while you have the opportunity to voice your feelings about things that in the future you may not have the opportunity to share your feelings about.

Appendix: Generic Forms for Advance Directives

Advance directive forms are available from a variety of sources. To get a free living will and a durable power of attorney for health care, ask your doctor, the admissions department at your local hospital, or your county or state medical society. You can also ask your attorney if he or she has forms, generally available for your state free of charge, or you can contact your state attorney general's office and ask how to obtain the forms that are accepted in your state.

In this Appendix we reproduce three advance directives: the durable power of attorney for health care, the living will and health care proxy, and the Values History. Either the durable power of attorney for health care or the health care proxy can be used to name a durable power of attorney agent. (You can choose the document whose wording and style you prefer.) The first two are generic documents. While these generic documents will be accepted in most circumstances, it is preferable to use your own state's designated forms (and in some states you may be *required* to do so by law). Please check your own state's version of the durable power of attorney for health care and the living will and health care proxy before using one of these generic forms.

If you have difficulty obtaining advance directive forms from the sources identified above, you can contact either of the following two organizations, both of which provide advance directives free of charge:

Choice In Dying	American Association of
200 Varick Street	Retired Persons
New York, N.Y. 10014	601 E Street, N.W.
212/366-5540	Washington, D.C. 20049
	202/728-4350

Durable Power of Attorney for Health Care

1. I, _____ , hereby appoint:

NAME   HOME ADDRESS

(   )
HOME TELEPHONE NUMBER

(   )
WORK TELEPHONE NUMBER

As my attorney-in-fact to make health-care decisions for me if I become unable to make my own health-care decisions. This gives my attorney-in-fact the power to grant, refuse, or withdraw consent on my behalf for any health-care service, treatment, or procedure, even though my death may ensue. My attorney-in-fact has the authority to talk to health-care personnel, get information, have access to medical records, and sign forms necessary to carry out these decisions. My attorney-in-fact also has authority to authorize my admission to or discharge from any hospital, nursing home, residential care, assisted living or similar facility or service, and to contract on my behalf for any health-care related service or facility (without my attorney-in-fact incurring personal financial liability for such contracts).

2. If the person named as my attorney-in-fact is not available or is unable to act as my attorney-in-fact, I appoint the following person(s) to serve in the order listed below:

a. _____
   NAME   HOME ADDRESS

   (   )
   HOME TELEPHONE NUMBER

   (   )
   WORK TELEPHONE NUMBER

b. _____
    NAME   HOME ADDRESS

(   ) _____

HOME TELEPHONE NUMBER

(   ) _____

WORK TELEPHONE NUMBER

3. With this document, I intend to create a durable power of attorney for health-care, which shall take effect upon and only during any period in which, in the opinion of two doctors, I am unable to make or communicate a choice regarding a particular health-care decision. My attorney-in-fact shall make health-care decisions as I direct below or as I make known to him or her in some other way. If my attorney-in-fact is unable to determine the choice I would want to make, then my attorney-in-fact shall make a choice for me based upon what my attorney-in-fact believes to be in my best interest.

a. STATEMENT OF DIRECTIVES CONCERNING LIFE-PROLONGING CARE, TREATMENT, SERVICES, AND PROCEDURES: (The directions herein apply to all forms of life-sustaining treatments which include but are not limited to mechanical ventilation, cardiopulmonary resuscitation, kidney dialysis, and artificial nutrition and hydration, unless otherwise limited in these directions).

_____

_____

_____

_____

_____

b. SPECIAL PROVISIONS AND LIMITATIONS: (These limitations and or provisions apply to specific types

130

of treatment that are inconsistent with my religious beliefs or unacceptable to me for any other reason, such as blood transfusions, convulsive therapy, amputations, psychosurgery, etc., and

_____

_____

_____

_____

_____

_____

4. To the extent that I am permitted by law to do so, I herewith nominate my attorney-in-fact to serve as my guardian, conservator and/or in any similar representative capacity. If I am not permitted by law to make a nomination, then I request in the strongest possible terms that any court consider this nomination.

5. No person who relies in good faith upon representations by my attorney-in-fact or alternate attorney-in-fact shall be liable to me, my estate, my heirs or assigns for recognizing the attorney-in-fact's authority.

6. The powers delegated under this power of attorney are separable, so that the invalidity of one or more powers shall not affect any others.

BY MY SIGNATURE I INDICATE THAT I UNDERSTAND THE PURPOSE AND EFFECT OF THIS DOCUMENT.

I sign my name to this form on _____
at: _____
    (ADDRESS)

_____
(SIGNATURE)

WITNESSES

I declare that the person who signed or acknowledged this document is personally known to me, that the person signed acknowledged this durable power of attorney for health care in my presence, and that the person appears to be of sound mind and under no duress, fraud, or undue influence. I am not the person appointed as attorney-in-fact by this document, nor am I the person's health-care provider or an employee of the person's health-care provider. I am not related to the person by blood, marriage or adoption, and to the best of my knowledge, I am not a creditor of the person, nor responsible for paying the person's health-care costs, nor entitled to any part of the person's estate under a will now existing or by operation of law.

First Witness:

Signature: _____

Home Address: _____

Print Name: _____

Date: _____

Second Witness:

Signature: _____

Home Address: _____

Print Name: _____

Date: _____

NOTARIZATION*

STATE OF _____) ss:

COUNTY OF _____)

*May be required in some states.

I, _____, a Notary Public in and for the State and County aforesaid, do hereby certify that _____, who is personally well known to me as the Principal, who executed the foregoing Durable Power of Attorney for Health Care in said State and County, and acknowledged that said Durable Power of Attorney for Health Care to be the Principal's free act and voluntary deed.

WITNESS my signature this _____ day of _____, 19____.

_____
NOTARY PUBLIC

Adapted from Barbara Mishkin, *A Matter of Choice: Planning Ahead for Health Care Decisions*, 2d ed. (Washington, D.C.: AARP, 1992). Courtesy Barbara Mishkin and AARP.

Living Will and Health Care Proxy

Death is a part of life. It is a reality like birth, growth and aging. I am using this advance directive to convey my wishes about medical care to my doctors and other people looking after me at the end of my life. It is called an advance directive because it gives instructions in advance about what I want to happen to me in the future. It expresses my wishes about medical treatment that might keep me alive. I want this to be legally binding.

If I cannot make or communicate decisions about my medical care, those around me should rely on this document for instructions about measures that could keep me alive.

I do not want medical treatment (including feeding and water by tube) that will keep me alive if:
- I am unconscious and there is no reasonable prospect that I will ever be conscious again (even if I am not going to die soon in my medical condition), *or*
- I am near death from an illness or injury with no reasonable prospect of recovery.

I do want medicine and other care to make me more comfortable and to take care of pain and suffering. I want this even if the pain medicine makes me die sooner.

I want to give some extra instructions: (*Here list any special instructions, e.g., some people fear being kept alive after a debilitating stroke. If you have wishes about this, or any other conditions, please write them here.*]

The legal language that follows is a health care proxy. It gives another person the power to make medical decisions for me.

I name _____ , who lives at

_____ ,

phone number _____ ,
to make medical decisions for me if I cannot make them
myself. This person is called a health care "surrogate,"
"agent," "proxy," or "attorney in fact." This power of attorney shall become effective when I become incapable of
making or communicating decisions about my medical
care. This means that this document stays legal when
and if I lose the power to speak for myself, for instance, if
I am in a coma or have Alzheimer's disease.

My health care proxy has power to tell others what my
advance directive means. This person also has power to
make decisions for me, based either on what I would
have wanted, or, if this is not known, on what he or she
thinks is best for me.

If my first choice health care proxy cannot or decides not
to act for me, I name _____ ,
address _____ ,
phone number _____ , as my
second choice.

I have discussed my wishes with my health care proxy,
and with my second choice if I have chosen to appoint a
second person. My proxy(ies) has(have) agreed to act for
me.

I have thought about this advance directive carefully. I
know what it means and want to sign it. I have chosen
two witnesses, neither of whom is a member of my family, nor will inherit from me when I die. My witnesses are
not the same people as those I named as my health care
proxies. I understand that this form should be notarized
if I name (a) health care proxy(ies).

Signature _____

Date _____

Address _____

Witness' signature _____

Witness' printed name _____

Address _____

Witness' signature _____

Witness' printed name _____

Address _____

Notary [to be used if proxy is appointed] _____

*Drafted and Distributed by Choice In Dying, Inc.—the National
Council for the Right to Die. Choice In Dying is a National not-for-
profit organization which works for the rights of patients at the end of
life. In addition to this generic advance directive, Choice In Dying dis-
tributes advance directives that conform to each state's specific legal
requirements and maintains a national Living Will Registry for completed documents.*

The Values History

Patient's name: _____

This Values History serves as a set of my specific value-based directives for various medical interventions. It is to be used in health care circumstances when I may be unable to voice my preferences. These directives shall be made a part of the medical record and shall be used as supplementary to my living will and/or durable power of attorney for health care if I am terminally ill or in a persistently vegetative state.

I. *Values Section*

There are several values important in decisions about end-of-life treatment and care. This section of the Values History invites you to identify your most important values.

A. Basic Life Values

Perhaps the most basic values in this context concern length of life versus quality of life. Which of the following two statements most accurately reflects your feelings and wishes? Write your initials and the date next to the number you choose.

_____ 1. I want to live as long as possible, regardless of the quality of life that I experience.

_____ 2. I want to preserve a good quality of life, even if this means that I may not live as long.

B. Quality-of-Life Values

There are many values that help us to define for ourselves the quality of life that we want to live. The following values appear to be those most frequently used to define quality of life. Review this list and circle the values that are most important to your definition of quality of life. Feel free to elaborate on any of the items in the list, and to add to the list any other values that are important to you.

1. I want to maintain my capacity to think clearly.
2. I want to feel safe and secure.
3. I want to avoid unnecessary pain and suffering.
4. I want to be treated with respect.
5. I want to be treated with dignity when I can no longer speak for myself.
6. I do not want to be an unnecessary burden on my family.
7. I want to be able to make my own decisions.
8. I want to experience a comfortable dying process.
9. I want to be with my loved ones before I die.
10. I want to leave good memories of me for my loved ones.
11. I want to be treated in accord with my religious beliefs and traditions.
12. I want respect shown for my body after I die.
13. I want to help others by making a contribution to medical education and research.
14. Other values or clarification of values above:

II. *Directives Section*

Some directives involve a simple yes or no decision. Others provide for the choice of a trial of intervention. Write your initials and the date next to the number for each directive you complete.

_____ 1. I want to undergo cardiopulmonary resuscitation.

____ YES

____ NO

Why?

_____ 2. I want to be placed on a ventilator.

____ YES

____ TRIAL for the TIME PERIOD OF _____ .

____ TRIAL to determine effectiveness using
reasonable medical judgment.

____ NO

Why?

_____ 3. I want to have an endotracheal tube used in
order to perform items 1 and 2.

____ YES

____ TRIAL for the TIME PERIOD OF _____ .

____ TRIAL to determine effectiveness using
reasonable medical judgment.

____ NO

Why?

_____ 4. I want to have total parenteral nutrition administered for my nutrition.

____ YES

____ TRIAL for the TIME PERIOD OF _____ .

____ TRIAL to determine effectiveness using
reasonable medical judgment.

____ NO

Why?

_____ 5. I want to have intravenous medication and hydration administered. Regardless of my decision, I understand that intravenous hydration to alleviate discomfort or pain medication will not be withheld from me if I so request them.

___ YES

___ TRIAL for the TIME PERIOD OF _____ .

___ TRIAL to determine effectiveness using reasonable medical judgment.

___ NO

Why?

_____ 6. I want to have all medications used for the treatment of my illness continued. Regardless of my decision, I understand that pain medication will continue to be administered including narcotic medications.

___ YES

___ TRIAL for the TIME PERIOD OF _____ .

___ TRIAL to determine effectiveness using reasonable medical judgment.

___ NO

Why?

_____ 7. I want to have nasogastric, gastrostomy, or other enteral feeding tubes introduced and administered for my nutrition.

___ YES

___ TRIAL for the TIME PERIOD OF _____ .

___ TRIAL to determine effectiveness using reasonable medical judgment.

___ NO

Why?

_____ 8. I want to be placed on a dialysis machine.

    _____ YES

    _____ TRIAL for the TIME PERIOD OF _____ .

    _____ TRIAL to determine effectiveness using reasonable medical judgment.

    _____ NO

Why?

_____ 9. I want to have an autopsy done to determine the cause(s) of my death.

    _____ YES

    _____ NO

Why?

_____ 10. I want to be admitted to the Intensive Care Unit.

    _____ YES

    _____ NO

Why?

_____ 11. *For a patient in a long-term care facility or for a patient receiving care at home who experiences a life-threatening change in health status:* I want 911 called in case of a medical emergency.

    _____ YES

    _____ NO

Why?

_____ 12. Other directives:

I consent to these directives after receiving honest disclosure of their implications, risks, and benefits from my physician, being free of constraints, and being of sound mind.

Signature: _____ Date: _____

Witness: _____

Witness: _____

13. Proxy Negation: I request that the following persons NOT be allowed to make decisions on my behalf in the event of my disability or incapacity:

_____

_____

_____

Signature: _____ Date: _____

Witness: _____

Witness: _____

14. Organ Donation:
(Insert here your state's version of the Organ Donor Card.)

15. Durable Power of Attorney for Health Care:
(Insert here your state's version of the durable power of attorney for health care.)

Adapted from David Doukas and Laurence McCullough, "The Values History: The Evaluation of the Patient's Values and Advance Directives," *Journal of Family Practice* 32 (February 1991): 145–53. Reprinted by permission of Appleton & Lange, Inc.

Index